Travel Medicine—Series I

Travel Medicine—Series I

Special Issue Editor
Larry Goodyer

MDPI • Basel • Beijing • Wuhan • Barcelona • Belgrade

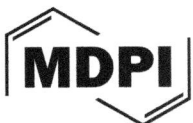

MDPI

Special Issue Editor
Larry Goodyer
De Montfort University
UK

Editorial Office
MDPI
St. Alban-Anlage 66
4052 Basel, Switzerland

This is a reprint of articles from the Special Issue published online in the open access journal *Pharmacy* (ISSN 2226-4787) from 2018 to 2019 (available at: https://www.mdpi.com/journal/pharmacy/special_issues/Travel_Medicine_I)

For citation purposes, cite each article independently as indicated on the article page online and as indicated below:

LastName, A.A.; LastName, B.B.; LastName, C.C. Article Title. *Journal Name* **Year**, *Article Number*, Page Range.

ISBN 978-3-03897-952-4 (Pbk)
ISBN 978-3-03897-953-1 (PDF)

Contents

About the Special Issue Editor

Larry Goodyer is a Professor of Pharmacy Practice and was formally the Head of the Leicester School of Pharmacy at De Montfort University UK. He has lectured and taught widely on travel medicine to both health professionals and the public and has been invited to address both national and international conferences on the subject, as well as appearing on television and radio broadcasts. Related research interests include methods for bite avoidance and medical supplies for overseas travel. He has been Chair of the British Global and Travel Health Association founding Chair of the Pharmacist Professional Group of the International Society of Travel Medicine. In addition, he is a Fellow of the Faculty of Travel Medicine at the RCPSG, Royal Geographic Society, and the International Society of Travel Medicine. More broadly in his capacity as a Professor of Pharmacy Practice, he has been involved in research and teaching on a wide range of issues related to the pharmacy profession. These include new roles for pharmacists such as prescribing and medicines optimisation.

pharmacy

MDPI

Editorial

Pharmacy and Travel Medicine: A Global Movement

Larry Goodyer

School of Pharmacy, De Montfort University, The Gateway, Leicester, LE1 9BH, UK; lgoodyer@dmu.ac.uk

Received: 15 April 2019; Accepted: 17 April 2019; Published: 24 April 2019

check for updates

This is the first special edition of a journal that has focused specifically on Pharmacy Practice and travel medicine. Pharmacist involvement in delivering travel health services is a relatively new phenomenon and if a call had gone out for similar publications just ten years ago, there would have been very few takers. Contained in this edition are a range of articles that examine current practice by pharmacists in delivering a travel medicine service, with some clearly describing how such services have developed. Some of these articles have been written by the committee members of the International Society of Travel Medicine (ISTM) Pharmacists Professional Group and I would encourage all pharmacists with an interest in this new discipline to join ISTM. Looking at these papers, there does seem to be a common thread in the process by which pharmacist involvement has grown so rapidly.

Undoubtably, there is a long and somewhat uncharted history whereby community-based pharmacists have offered informal advice and support to the travelling public. Many will visit a pharmacy before departure for travel-related medicines and other health products, whereby a pharmacist might be approached for advice. However, it is only recently that they have offered full services that include consultations and vaccinations. In many countries, the development has begun with changes in legislation and policy to allow pharmacists to administer influenza vaccines as part of national immunization programmes. Alongside this has been the introduction of mechanisms that allow pharmacists to supply prescription-only medicine, either by special protocols, gaining limited prescribing authority, or in some cases, full prescribing authority. It was not long after the introduction of influenza pharmacy programmes that pharmacists then began to offer other vaccination services, including those associated with travel. In some regions, community pharmacists can also offer prescription items for travel, including antimalarials and antibiotics, as prescribers themselves or under protocol. Even community pharmacy premises have undergone changes, with most now having a consultation room in which such clinical services can be delivered. It will not be long before the pharmacist becomes as much associated with the consultation area as the dispensary.

As always, with such rapid changes, there could be potential challenges and issues that may need be addressed. An important consideration is the further training of pharmacists to deliver such services. The immunization technique is not taught as part of the preregistration/undergraduate curriculum in all regions where pharmacists undertake such activities. Robust training and assessment of these skills should be undertaken post-registration and competence should be updated regularly. In addition, Travel Medicine is becoming a specialty in its own right and pharmacists should be prepared to engage with the necessary education and training required to deliver a safe and effective service.

There is a potential issue concerning pharmacists who do not give various vaccines on a regular basis in terms of maintaining their competence. Further, there is an important distinction between offering a vaccination supply and administration service and a full travel health service. The latter requires a comprehensive risk assessment of travelers and constructing a management plan that could take a considerable amount of time for those with complex itineraries and/or special needs. This implies not only a call on the pharmacist's time from other duties, but a higher level of training and competence. It could be argued that the vast majority of the traveling public do not require such comprehensive

Pharmacy **2019**, *7*, 39

consultations, e.g., they go on lower-risk short holidays in resorts where perhaps one or two vaccines have been recommended, and the pharmacist may not need extensive further training. However, those travelers at a greater risk should ideally be referred to a more highly trained and experienced pharmacist or another health professional. It is uncertain as to whether such referrals will take place in the community pharmacy environment.

To date, there does seem to be a good level of satisfaction amongst users of pharmacy services and perhaps a continued rise in provision will raise awareness amongst the traveling public to seek advice. Further work is needed to identify the training needs, models of delivery, and effectiveness of this new pharmacy activity.

Conflicts of Interest: The author declare no conflict of interest.

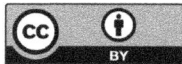

pharmacy

MDPI

Article

Pharmacy Travel Health Services in Canada: Experience of Early Adopters

Doug Thidrickson [1] and Larry Goodyer [2,*]

[1] Access Fort Garry, Winnipeg Regional Health Authority, Winnipeg, MB R3T 6E8, Canada;
    dthidrickson@wrha.mb.ca
[2] School of Pharmacy, De Montfort University, Leicester LE1 9BH, UK
*   Correspondence: lgoodyer@dmu.ac.uk; Tel.: +44-01162506100

Received: 15 April 2019; Accepted: 23 April 2019; Published: 27 April 2019

check for
updates

Abstract: Since 2007, community pharmacists in Canada have become increasingly involved in delivering Travel Health services, including the recommendation and administration of vaccines. This qualitative scoping survey examines some of the activities and opinions of those early pharmacist adopters delivering these services. A Survey Monkey free text questionnaire was emailed to pharmacists who were involved in delivering travel medicine services. 21 pharmacists responding represented seven Canadian provinces. Only 5 pharmacists estimated that they were seeing five or more patients a week on average. Amongst the challenges they faced the most quoted was lack of time when running a busy pharmacy (62%) a lack of prescribing authority, (52%), and lack of access to public health vaccines (52%). 'Word of mouth' was widely quoted as a means of developing the service, indicating a good patient satisfaction. Also expressed were the advantages of convenience in terms of being a 'one stop shop', ease of billing to insurance companies and convenient appointment times. There are a number of challenges which are still to be faced which may be resolved by further legislation allowing access to public health vaccines and more widespread prescribing rights. The relatively low level of consultations reported by some is of concern if those pharmacists are to maintain competence.

Keywords: travel medicine; community pharmacy; vaccination; Canada

1. Introduction

In the last decade, Canadian pharmacists have taken an increasing role providing travel health services [1,2]. Many factors have influenced this trend including the rise in international travellers, expanding scope of practice, changes in government funding and lack of timely access to travel health services. Traditionally, these services were only provided by specialty clinics. In addition to specialty clinics, it is currently provided by primary care providers, public health nurses and pharmacists; with or without training in this field of study. Pharmacists are in a unique position to heighten traveller awareness of the benefits of pretravel preparedness and increase accessibility and convenience of travel health services.

Pharmacists have seen their scope of practice expand dramatically over the past 20 years including the administration of vaccines and prescribing. In an effort to encourage greater vaccination rates and based on the successes of expanding scope in other countries, provincial pharmacy regulators pushed for administration of vaccines by pharmacists. In 2019, pharmacists in all Canadian provinces now have the authority to administer vaccines by injection with the exception of Quebec. Prescribing by pharmacists has also expanded. Alberta pioneered the Advanced Prescribing Authority (APA) program in 2007 to allow pharmacists with the APA designation to prescribe for almost any medication, including vaccines and medications to reduce travel health risks. Other provinces such as Prince Edward Island,

New Brunswick, Newfoundland and Nova Scotia recognize prescribing of some additional travel vaccines with additional training, although not necessarily in travel health. It is encouraging to see the ISTM Certificate of Travel Health increasingly recognized by provincial regulatory pharmacy authorities as a requirement for prescribing authority in travel health. Manitoba, Saskatchewan and Nova Scotia are provinces that have current or proposed regulations to support this prescribing authority. The Canadian Pharmacy Association [3] has produced a by Province/Territory overview which describes where authority for pharmacists to administer vaccines, including those for travel, is currently legislated. This shows considerable variation amongst regions as to what is permitted. Similarly prescribing authority or the ability to supply collaboratively prescription medicines also varies greatly across regions.

This is the first national Canadian survey that demonstrates how pharmacists maximizing their scope of practice can improve awareness and convenience of travel health services.

The aim of this study is to gain a view of the personal experience of the first adopters amongst pharmacists who are delivering a full travel health service, which involves risk-assessment, administration of vaccines, education to reduce travel risks and post travel follow-up.

2. Methods

This is a qualitative study that attempted to describe the experiences of pharmacists delivering travel health services. The aim being to do an environmental scan on three broad aspects of service amongst a sample of early adopters. Data was captured via a 6-point questionnaire designed using the Survey Monkey software that in the main comprised of free text boxes posing three broad questions:

1. Identify the challenges you experienced providing travel health services. For this participants were asked to select from four potential challenges they had faced introducing their service, with a free text box to describe these challenges or any other that had been encountered
2. Can you provide examples where offering this service increased awareness of the benefits of pharmacy-based travel services?
3. Can you provide examples where offering this service increased convenience for the traveller?

The other questions included indicating the province they were located, a tick box for the range of travel health services offered and the number of consultations on average they conducted per week.

Being a qualitative exercise a purposive sampling approach was taken, the aim being to have at least one pharmacist represented in each province. An invitation to take part was posted, with an email link to the questionnaire, to all pharmacies in the Amenity Healthcare Network at the time (32 stores), which are mainly independent pharmacies located in Western Canada. An invitation to take part was also posted on the International Society of Travel Medicine Pharmacist Professional Group Forum. In addition those pharmacies outside the network known to the author to be active in providing Travel Medicines services were invited.

The survey was open from 18 March 2018 to 29 April 2018. A total of 21 responses were received.

No information by which a pharmacist could by identified was gathered and implied consent to participate was assumed if a pharmacist submitted the questionnaire. For this reason and because it is a non-interventionary study ethical approval was not sought.

A thematic approach was adopted in the analysis of the free text responses.

3. Results

A total of 21 pharmacists responded to the survey and 20 of these stated that in their travel Health service the Pharmacist provides risk assessments, vaccinations and education to reduce travel health risks. One pharmacist did not answer this question. Respondent 10described that:

Current scope does not allow for schedule 1 injections such as yellow fever, Japanese encephalitis, and rabies. I am told this will be remedied by our college in the future. (Pharmacist 1, Nova Scotia)

Table 1 one refers to the Canadian province in which the pharmacist is practicing and their estimated average number of travel health consultations per week. The province of Saskatchewan , Newfoundland/Labrador and Canadian Territories and Quebec were not represented in the sample but may be amongst the four where the pharmacist did not provide their area of jurisdiction. Pharmacists did report on the seasonality of numbers of consultations.

Table 1. Jurisdiction of Pharmacies, number of travel consultations and potential challenges.

Question	N (%)
Province/Jurisdiction	
British Columbia	3 (14)
Alberta	5 (24)
Manitoba	2 (10)
Ontario	4 (19)
New Brunswick	1 (5)
Nova Scotia	1 (5)
Prince Edward Island	1 (5)
Not stated	4 (19)
Consultations per week	
<1	7 (33)
1–2	1 (5)
3–4	5 (24)
5–6	2 (10)
7–8	1 (5)
>8	2 (10)
Not stated	3 (14)

3.1. Challenges to The Service

The numbers reporting various challenges to delivering the service are shown in Table 2. These were supported and expanded upon by free text comments made by nine of the pharmacists.

Table 2. Challenges experienced.

Challenge	N (%)
Lack of prescribing authority	11 (52)
Integration into busy pharmacy	13 (62)
Access to public health vaccines *	11 (52)
Maintaining competence	4 (19)
None stated	2 (10)

*. Routine vaccines (Tdap, HPV etc.) are offered free of charge to eligible Canadians. However, if these are accessed through a pharmacy, the pharmacy is not reimbursed and the patient will need to pay for the product PLUS a dispensing fee. A known exception is Manitoba where there is free access to some routine vaccine products (no cost to pharmacy or patient) and the provincial government pays a dispensing fee for five routine adult vaccinations.

Resources and time were identified as challenges to providing a service that met client expectations.

At the moment it is owner operated so appointments are scheduled during non-dispensing hours. It would be challenging for a staff pharmacist to run without more resources (Pharmacist 1, Nova Scotia)

When i have to write the rx, type them, fill them, check them it takes time in the middle of the consult leaving the patient to twiddle their thumbs for 15–20 min (Pharmacist 1, New Brunswick)

One pharmacist felt that high expectations of an instant response as for other types of consultations could not be met with this service.

Patients are accustomed to contacting their pharmacists and getting an answer quickly… expectation that it is the same with travel consult… By the way I am going to Nicaragua, and expecting an answer now. (Pharmacist 1 Ontario)

Competition for services from other pharmacies and clinics was also seen as a challenge by two pharmacists. Only one mentioned direct lack of support by other physicians.

Increased competition, even from pharmacies with no ISTM-certified staff; other responsibilities of store ownership (Pharmacist 1, Alberta)

Vaccine backorders, prescribers insisting patients go to a "real" travel clinic (Province not stated)

A backorder refers to non-availability of the item in stock.

In those provinces where vaccination could be provided free by doctor services or travel services billed for a related and eligible medical condition, this was seen to be a barrier for increased pharmacy involvement.

Patients feel professional fees are unreasonable and refuse to pay, since they feel they can see their doctor and receive vaccinations and services for free. (Province not stated)

One pharmacist felt a lack of access to appropriate resources was an issue.

The ease in getting vaccination histories could be dramatically improved if travel health Pharmacists would be allowed to access MIMS etc. (Pharmacist 1, Manitoba)

MIMS refers to the provincial vaccination records for the patient.

3.2. Convenience of The Service

From the free text responses concerning opinions on whether a pharmacy travel health service might have any benefits in terms of convenience to the traveller, all were able to cite specific examples from their own practice. In addition, in this section pharmacists chose to articulate a range of other clinical benefits they thought their service offered. These were categorised under four themes.

3.2.1. A One Stop Shop

The convenience of being able to access the services required in one place.

Assessment, Prescription, Dispensing and Administration at one spot (Pharmacist 2, Alberta)

Although not being able to prescribe medicines limited this to some extent.

Travellers can get most of their travel health needs attended to in a one-stop shop, with the exception of requiring a physician's Rx for antimalarials and antibiotics, etc. All vaccines can be prescribed and administered by the pharmacist, and travel health kits sold with OTC items. (Pharmacist 1, British Columbia)

A pharmacist who could prescribe pointed out the benefits to patients.

We offer a 1-stop travel assessment where patients can have the assessment done, have appropriate meds prescribed, have prescriptions filled, have vaccines administered, and be counseled on travel meds in 1 single visit. Since our pharmacists are authorized to prescribe, we do not have to wait to hear back from their family prescriber to approve our recommendations. (Pharmacist 3, Alberta)

Family prescriber refers to the General Practitioner.

3.2.2. Convenience of Appointments

Pharmacists gave examples of how their opening hours were convenient to clients and perhaps more flexible than other types of clinics.

Quicker and more convenient access to appointments has been a huge opportunity for my patients. I can book Monday to Sunday at almost any time and generally can meet people for next day up to 2 weeks later (Pharmacist 2, Manitoba)

Over the past 6 months, probably 30%-40% of my consultations would be considered short notice that probably was the only way the traveler would have been seen. i.e., by a Pharmacist such as myself offering the convenience. (Pharmacist 1, Manitoba)

Evening appointments, allow patients to follow up by email if they have further questions

Adjudicating insurance on the spot is helpful for patients. More accessible hours than many travel clinics. (Pharmacist 2, British Columbia)

Such convenience was felt to be limited for those who did not have prescribing rights but still offered an advantage.

We can usually see patients within a couple of days. In BC we do not have prescriptive authority so have to wait to have family physician sign off on medications required but can do vaccines and consult in one visit (Pharmacist 3, British Columbia)

As we cannot prescribe, the patient still must either meet with the doctor OR wait for the doctor to respond to (and accept) our recommendations. However, the ability to dispense and inject vaccines in one visit to the pharmacy saves the patient a return trip to the doctor for injections. Additionally patients are made to wait at the doctor's office for vaccinations, we can usually fit patients in right away. Patients can pick up all OTC needs in the same pharmacy visit as well. (Pharmacist 2, Ontario)

3.2.3. Paying through an Insurance Plan

For the pharmacist to be able to arrange paying for medication and services through an insurance plan during the decision-making process did seem to be an important area of convenience to the patient and this was described by five of the pharmacist.

One stop service is highly convenient for the customer Ability to direct bill plan (Pharmacist 4, Alberta)

The direct bill plan refers to an invoice sent electronically sent to the drug plan company, who will pay for 80% or 100% of the cost of drug plus dispensing fee, via an intermediary.

Being able to bill their insurance plan has also been a benefit for the patients. (Pharmacist 2, Manitoba)

Pharmacists can bill insurance plans vs travel clinics generally do not. (Pharmacist 1, New Brunswick)

3.2.4. Clinical Benefits

One pharmacist mentioned specifically the specialist knowledge of the pharmacist.

Pharmacist can administer injections and prescribe and provide travel meds at the same visit. Also, pharmacist will assess interactions with current med list. Taking interactions and allergies in consideration, the right meds will be prescribed (Pharmacist 5, Alberta)

Some specific clinical outcomes of pharmacist's consultations were also described.

Easier for a customer to consult his/her pharmacist as the pharmacist knows his medical conditions, med list and can administer his injections and provide travel meds right after the consult (Pharmacist 5, Alberta)

I have had several patients return to me after receiving a travel consultation to get their flu shot, prescribe for a minor ailment or perform a different assessment (e.g., smoking cessation) (Pharmacist 3, Alberta)

3.3. Raising Awareness

All of the Pharmacists could describe ways in which awareness of the service had been raised. The comments fell into passive and proactive themes.

3.3.1. Passive

Most mentioned that clients came to consults due to word of mouth often by other clients pleased with the service.

We get a lot of returning customers, and a lot of word-of-mouth referrals (Pharmacist 1, Prince Edward Island)

A number mentioned in addition referrals and a good level of cooperation with local physicians and other health centres.

We have had some success with word-of-mouth between returning customers and also with family physicians in the area (Pharmacist 2, Ontario)

Collaboration with Family Dr, Business cards given out in community to market the service (Pharmacist 1, New Brunswick)

I have received many referrals from travelers that I have provided consultations to in the past as well as from physicians that I have personally consulted as well. (Pharmacist 1 Manitoba)

In January 2018, our health unit is no longer offering the travel health services. Therefor the health unit is referring travelers to some of the pharmacy in our community. (Pharmacist 1, Ontario)

3.3.2. Proactive Marketing

As well as returning clients and word of mouth, pharmacists also proactively advertised services and identified potential clients using the pharmacy.

Many regular customers travel frequently, and because our pharmacy has only been offering travel consultation for about a year, we are starting to market this when we pick up on certain flags—i.e., customer asks for early fills for travel, customer looking at brochures on travel health, OTC questions, and direct requests for vaccine advice. Many customers now aware that we offer this and referrals to their neighbours and friends is starting. (Pharmacist 1, British Columbia)

Other marketing material was reported as being used, included brochures and posters which were distributed both within the pharmacy and in other relevant locations in the community.

Created brochures and posters to display travel services offered, sent them to local travel agents and doctors and hung them in pharmacy (Pharmacist 3, Ontario)

Two pharmacists described being invited to give presentations in a variety of settings.

I've been invited to present about travel health to a community travel group, which increased their awareness of both potential health risks, as well as how to access pre travel advise. It has increased my colleague's awareness of being able to provide this service, which has improved access. My staff talk about it more with customers, improving access. I've also been invited by the school of pharmacy to give a lecture on travel infections. (Pharmacist 2, Manitoba)

We have done a lunch and learn at our local medical office which our physicians found informative and have had referrals from them. (Pharmacist 3, British Columbia)

4. Discussion

The range of responses is to some extent a reflection of the variation in legislation across the provinces in Canada limiting the type of service that pharmacists can offer [3]. In some provinces for instance the full range of travel vaccines cannot be offered and in others antimalarial prophylaxis cannot be supplied without a physician's prescription. Lack of prescribing authority was seen as a major challenge to developing services. In time though it is likely that such variations will disappear. The other major challenge was integrating the service into the pharmacist's other duties in a busy environment. As Canadian community pharmacists take on more clinical roles their working practices, in particular in medicine dispensing and distribution, will need to be delegated to other pharmacy staff or centralized systems. This has been recognized in other countries such as the UK where community pharmacy has been developing in a similar way. [4] Although a study in 2015 conducted in a single medium sized pharmacy chain in Alberta did indicate that pharmacists had a low baseline knowledge and poor confidence in their abilities to deliver a travel health service, this may well have changed in that none volunteered such issues regarding challenges [5].

Only five of the pharmacies estimated that they achieved above the five minimum per week recommended by the **Committee to Advise on Tropical Medicine and Travel** (CATMAT) Guidelines for the Practice of Travel Medicine [6] in order to maintain a good level of competence. The question did remind the pharmacists of the Current CATMAT guidelines. This low activity may be due to having a recently introduced service which would take time to build numbers. Most observed a very seasonal nature of the demand making it difficult to provide weekly estimates.

The pharmacists described a range of examples of proactive marketing and promotion of services. Some also anecdotally reported that services were promoted and recommended by patients through word of mouth with a growing base of returning customers. By implication this would indicate a broad satisfaction with the pharmacist provided travel health services, as found by Houle [2]. In the article by Zimmer [7] an argument was made against a market-driven approach for the provision of travel health services in Canada as might be provided by pharmacists. The implication was that patients may be coerced into unnecessary vaccinations. This did not appear as issue in this study though this question was not directly addressed and there were no reports of patient dissatisfaction. However, this was not asked directly so could be viewed as an area of bias in the study and needs to be explored in future work.

It appeared that there were examples where local doctors and practices were welcoming of the pharmacy services and willing to refer patients as well as inviting meetings/presentations from the pharmacists. There was only one example of hostility by practices to the service, but no direct question was asked regarding the relationship between pharmacies and other local clinics delivering Travel Health Services.

Pharmacist identified that the ease with which appointments could be obtained at times that best suited the patients as a major advantage of their service. In those provinces where pharmacist prescribing was legislated, they could provide a 'one stop shop' for traveller's health needs. Ease of billing for services to insurers was also reported as an advantage. The financial aspect of uptake of immunization is important as access to insurance, the individual's overall financial flexibility, the burden of drug cost on the individual's budget and the importance of the drug from the individual's perspective all influence cost-related non-adherence [8]. Pharmacists also identified a number of clinical benefits to patient consulting with a pharmacist such as related to potential drug or disease interactions and offering other opportunistic health related services.

Future work could usefully explore some of the themes identified in this informal scoping exercise to identify the models of practice that have been implemented by pharmacists in delivering their travel health services. Such models are likely to depend to a great extent on the legislative authority in place to permit prescribing of medicine and administration of vaccines related to travel medicine. Further formal qualitative investigation, which employ in depth interviewing techniques, might also explore both the benefits and challenges experienced by pharmacists delivering these services and their opinions how these might be best overcome.

Internationally there have been studies that have shown good acceptance for pharmacy-based vaccination programmes [9] and some limited work that pharmacist delivered travel health services have positive benefits [10–12]. It does appear from the present study that there is good satisfaction amongst patients regarding the travel health services they receive form the pharmacist, as was also identified in a single travel clinic in Alberta [2]. But further work is needed to more clearly describe the outcomes of these services.

5. Limitations

The original intent of the survey was an informal environment scan of Canadian pharmacy-based travel services. The survey was not optimized for survey response rate or national representation. It is also recognized that the study and conclusions are based upon written free text statements by the respondents that could not be further explored as would have been the case in an interview based qualitative study. There may be a bias in respondents being the most proactive in establishing travel health services, though it was the intension to gain the views of the early enthusiasts. In addition, some provinces had only a single pharmacist responding. In general, questions tended to ask pharmacists to look for specific positive aspects of their service and only one question, although well answered, asked pharmacists for negative aspects.

6. Conclusions

Overall the respondents report a positive picture at this early stage of introduction of pharmacy based travel health services. The key benefit that pharmacist feel they bring, and one appreciated by patients is 'Convenience' be that through ease of appointments, offering a 'one stop shop' or the billing process. They were actively promoting their services though many were still seeing relatively few patients. Challenges of lack of time and in some province's limitations in prescribing authority were identified.

Author Contributions: For research articles with several authors, a short paragraph specifying their individual contributions must be provided. The following statements should be used "conceptualization, D.T.; methodology, D.T.; formal analysis, L.G.; investigation, D.T.; data curation, D.T. writing—original draft preparation, L.G.; writing—review and editing, D.T.; project administration, D.T.

Funding: This research received no external funding.

Conflicts of Interest: The authors declare no conflict of interest.

References

1. Bui, Y.G.; Kuhn, S.; Sow, M.; McCarthy, A.E.; Geduld, J.; Milord, F. The changing landscape of travel health services in Canada. *J. Travel Med.* **2018**, *25*. [CrossRef]
2. Houle, S.K.D.; Bascom, C.S.; Rosenthal, M.M. Clinical outcomes and satisfaction with a pharmacist-managed travel clinic in Alberta, Canada. *Travel Med. Infect. Dis.* **2018**, *23*, 21–26. [CrossRef] [PubMed]
3. Canadian Pharmacists Association. Pharmacists' Expanded Scope of Practice. Available online: https://www.pharmacists.ca/pharmacy-in-canada/scope-of-practice-canada/ (accessed on 11 April 2019).
4. Richardson, E.; Pollock AMRichardson, E.; Pollock, A.M. Community pharmacy: Moving from dispensing to diagnosis and treatment. *BMJ* **2010**, *340*. [CrossRef] [PubMed]
5. Bascom, C.; Rosenthal, M.M.; Houle, S.K.D. Are Pharmacists Ready for a Greater Role in Travel Health? An Evaluation of the Knowledge and Confidence in Providing Travel Health Advice of Pharmacists Practicing in a Community Pharmacy Chain in Alberta, Canada. *J. Travel Med.* **2015**, *22*, 99–104. [CrossRef] [PubMed]

6. Guidelines for the Practice of Travel Medicine (CATMAT). Available online: https://www.canada.ca/en/public-health/services/reports-publications/canada-communicable-disease-report-ccdr/monthly-issue/2009-35/guidelines-practice-travel-medicine.html (accessed on 11 April 2019).
7. Zimmer, R. Competing visions for travel health services in Canada. *J. Travel Med.* **2018**, *25*. [CrossRef] [PubMed]
8. Goldsmith, L.J.; Kolhatkar, A.; Popowich, D.; Holbrook, A.M.; Morgan, S.G.; Law, M.R. Understanding the patient experience of cost-related non-adherence to prescription medications through typology development and application. *Soc. Sci. Med.* **2017**, *194*, 51–59. [CrossRef] [PubMed]
9. Houle, S.K. Pharmacy travel health services: Current perspectives and future prospects. *Integr. Pharm. Res. Pract.* **2017**, *7*, 13–20. [CrossRef] [PubMed]
10. Durham, M.J.; Goad, J.A.; Neinstein, L.S.; Lou, M. A comparison of pharmacist travelhealth specialists' versus primary care providers' recommendations for travel-related medications, vaccinations and patient compliance in a college health setting. *J. Travel Med.* **2010**, *18*, 20–25. [CrossRef] [PubMed]
11. Hess, K.M.; Dai, C.; Garner, B.; Law, A.V. Measuring outcomes of a pharmacist-run travel health clinic located in an independent community pharmacy. *J. Am. Pharm. Assoc.* **2010**, *50*, 174–180. [CrossRef] [PubMed]
12. Tran, D.; Gatewood, S.; Moczygemba, L.R.; Stanley, D.D.; Goode, J.V. Evaluating health outcomes following a pharmacist-provided comprehensive pretravel health clinic in a supermarket pharmacy. *J. Am. Pharm. Assoc.* **2015**, *55*, 143–152. [CrossRef] [PubMed]

pharmacy

MDPI

Article

Australian Pharmacists' Perceptions and Practices in Travel Health

Ian M. Heslop [1,*], Richard Speare [2], Michelle Bellingan [1] and Beverley D. Glass [1]

[1] Pharmacy, College of Medicine and Dentistry, James Cook University, Townsville 4811, Australia;
     michelle.bellingan@jcu.edu.au (M.B.); beverley.glass@jcu.edu.au (B.D.G.)
[2] Public Health and Tropical Medicine, College of Public Health, Medical and Veterinary Sciences,
     James Cook University, Townsville 4811, Australia; richard.speare@jcu.edu.au
*   Correspondence: ian.heslop@jcu.edu.au

Received: 9 August 2018; Accepted: 20 August 2018; Published: 22 August 2018

Abstract: Worldwide, pharmacists are playing an increasing role in travel health, although legislation and funding can dictate the nature of this role, which varies from country to country. The aim of this study was to explore the current and potential future practices in travel health for pharmacists in Australia, as well as the perceived barriers, including training needs, for the provision of services. A survey was developed and participation was sought from a representative sample of Australian pharmacists, with descriptive statistics calculated to summarise the frequency of responses. A total of 255 participants, predominantly female (69%), below 50 years (75%) and registered less than 30 years completed the survey. Although over two-thirds (68%) provided travel-related advice in their current practice, the frequency of advice provision was low (less than 2 travellers per week) and limited to responding to travellers questions. Although Australian pharmacists are currently unable to administer travel vaccines and prescription only medications without prescription, they still consider travel health to be an appropriate role and that their clients would seek travel health advice from pharmacies if offered. Currently, key roles for Australian pharmacists are advising travellers who do not seek advice from other practitioners, reinforcing the advice of other health practitioners and referring travellers needing vaccinations and antimalarials. In order to expand these services, the barriers of workload, time, staffing and the need for training in travel health need to be addressed. In summary, the travel health services provided by pharmacies in Australia still have a way to go before they match the services offered by pharmacies in some other countries, however Australian pharmacist are keen to further develop their role in this area.

Keywords: pharmacist; travel health; Australia

1. Introduction

International travel is on the increase, especially to destinations in Asia, Africa and other emerging economies and the associated health risks of these destinations highlights the need for pre-travel health consultations [1,2]. Despite this, many travellers do not obtain pre-travel health advice before travelling overseas and, those who do, mainly seek advice from their general practitioner, a travel health clinic or specialist, or the internet [3–7]. Pharmacies do offer some travel health services, although the type and level of these services may vary, with pharmacy-run travel health services enjoying limited patronage. However, it has been suggested that pharmacies are perhaps an underutilised resource and that their accessibility, convenient location and the trust placed in pharmacists by the public make them an appropriate source of pre-travel health information [8–10].

A comprehensive assessment, analysis of risk and tailored counselling are all important for the pharmacist to deliver evidenced–based pre-travel health consultations. Current practice for pharmacists in travel health may vary significantly from country to country and can be attributed to legislative differences which may often not allow pharmacists, for example in South Africa, to prescribe or dispense medications without prescriptions as well as administer travel vaccines [11]. However, the scope of practice for South African pharmacists has expanded as a result of the down scheduling of some antimalarial drugs [11]. Similarly, within the UK, changes in the legislation providing pharmacists with a wider scope of practice to supply some prescription only medications combined with a 5% increase in the number of Britons travelling aboard has led to pharmacists having a greater role within a nationally funded travel health service [12]. Some of these current initiatives have been well received in the UK, with patients reporting that a pharmacy-run travel health service both met their needs and provided value for money [13].

Bascom et al. however reported that the overall confidence in providing travel health advice in a group of pharmacists surveyed in Alberta, Canada was low, with incomplete knowledge possibly impacting their ability to this provide advice. Although this study was limited by the sample size, it is suggested that this barrier could be addressed by training programs, both at undergraduate level and with continuing professional education [14]. The findings of this study were revisited by Houle, who found that pharmacists were confident in areas most commonly seen in community pharmacy practice, with 67% confident that they had the ability to source the required information. This again highlights the need for inclusion of travel health into university curricula to expand the scope of practice to include these new practice opportunities.

Houle, in a review on current and future prospects for travel health services, indicated the role that pharmacist have been playing in ensuring the cold chain for vaccinations has placed them in a good position to extend their scope of practice from administering just the influenza vaccine to travel vaccines [2]. This has already been adopted in some Canadian jurisdictions [2]. There are a number of different pharmacist prescribing models across the UK, USA and Canada, with pharmacists in all countries traditionally providing non-prescription drugs for traveller's diarrhoea, motion sickness and sun and insect bite protection [2,10,12–17]. The well-established medication documentation systems of pharmacies could also play a role in assisting patients to maintain documentation on their vaccination history and while travel health consultations focus largely on infectious diseases, the impact of non-infectious causes of morbidity and motility during travel cannot be overemphasised and this again presents pharmacists with an opportunity for which they are already trained [12–17].

The aim of this study was thus to examine both the current practices and opportunities for future practice of Australian pharmacists in the provision of travel health services. Their views regarding some of the barriers to implementation of these services and the need for training will also be explored.

2. Materials and Methods

2.1. Study Design and Participants

This study involved a cross-sectional survey of Australian pharmacists. The questionnaire was formatted into an electronic e-survey using SurveyMonkey®. Invitations to participate and hyperlinks to the questionnaire and participant information leaflet, were then e-mailed to all members of the Pharmaceutical Society of Australia in a weekly newsletter. In addition, the self-completion questionnaire was also formatted into a postal survey using Microsoft Word® and posted to a representative, stratified sample of 600 Australian community pharmacies. This sample was drawn from the estimated 7600 pharmacy businesses listed in the then current Yellow Pages® Business Directory for Australia using a systematic random sampling technique, ensuring a representative sample. The e-survey was open for a 6-week period from late March 2009 and the postal survey was open for a 6-week period from early May 2009.

2.2. Questionnaire Design and Testing

A self-completion questionnaire, consisting of a combination of 44 multiple choice questions (MCQs), multiple answer questions (MAQs), open answer and rating scale questions (using 5 point Likert scales) was designed to meet the objectives of the study. Questions were divided into 3 main sections; Demographics, Current travel health services and Perceptions of current and future travel services. To ensure the validity and reliability and to reduce bias and to allow comparison with other studies, some of the questions used in the self-completion questionnaire were based on similar questions used in other surveys [18,19]. In addition, before the questionnaire was distributed, it was pre-tested by a group of 5 pharmacists for understanding, readability and to ensure a timely completion. Only minor grammatical changes were then made prior to distribution.

2.3. Data Analysis

The responses to the e-survey and postal surveys were entered into Microsoft Excel® spreadsheets and the IBM® SPSS Statistics Package® (Version 22) was used for statistical analyses.

2.4. Ethical Considerations

Ethical approval for the study was granted by the James Cook University Human Research and Ethics Committee (Approval No: H3182) and approval to send a postal survey to the community pharmacies was obtained from the Survey Approval Program of the Pharmacy Guild of Australia (Approval No: 755).

3. Results

3.1. Respondent Characteristics

A total of 255 participants completed the survey. Participants were predominantly female (69%, 176/255), below the age of 50 years (74.5%, 190/255) and registered less than 30 years as a pharmacist (80.4%, 205/255). Most resided in metropolitan areas or capital cities (77.3%, 197/255) and were working in full-time positions (69.4%, 177/255), predominantly in community pharmacy (78.4%, 121/255). The majority of respondents had standard entry level pharmacy qualifications (82.7%, 211/255) and some had additional postgraduate qualifications including 9.8% (25/225) with postgraduate certificates, 6.7% (17/255) with a Master's degree and 0.8% (2/255) with doctorates. All Australian States and Territories were represented in the sample.

3.2. Current Practices

Over two-thirds of respondents (68.2%, 174/255) provided travel-related advice or services. However, their travel health workload was generally low, with the majority advising less than two travellers per week (69%, 120/174) and/or spending less than one hour per week on the provision of these services (83.9%, 146/174). The respondents reported that they commonly advise Australian travellers aged either below the age of 30 (56.9%, 99/174) or above the age of 50 (47.7%, 83/174), travelling for leisure (98.9%, 172/174), business (51.2%, 89/174) or were visiting friends and relatives (51.7%, 90/174) and to destinations in mainly in Southeast Asia (92%, 160/174), Western Europe (54%, 94/174) or Oceania (28.2%, 49/174) regions.

When questioned about the type and level of travel health service offered, over a third of respondents (34.5%, 60/174) reported that they only responded to travellers' questions and did not perform formal pre-travel health risk assessments, although 64.5% (112/174) of respondents reported that they did ask the traveller questions about their itinerary and medical history. Only 2 respondents (1.1%) completed full, formal pre-travel health risk assessments for their clients. In addition, respondents were asked to rate how often they counselled travellers on a range of 26 recommended travel health topics using a 5-point Likert scale. The mean ratings were calculated and are presented in Table 1. The majority of respondents (59.8%, 104/174) reported that they counselled travellers using a combination of written and verbal information and a similar number reported that they used generic drug information resources such as the Australian Medicines Handbook and the Australian Immunisation Handbook to respond to travellers' questions, whereas few reported that they used more travel-specific websites such as MASTA (34.5%, 60/174) and Travax (19%, 33/174).

Table 1. Average ratings for how frequently respondents advise travellers about common travel-related health topics (In order. Top 10 topics shaded) (n = 174).

Counselling Topic	Average Rating (Scale 1–5)
Treatment of diarrhoeal diseases	4.2
Prevention of mosquito and other insect bites	4.2
Safe food and water consumption	4.0
The need for antimalarial chemoprophylaxis	3.9
Travelling with medications for chronic conditions	3.9
Vaccinations needed for the traveller's destination	3.8
Risk and prevention of deep vein thrombosis	3.3
Dealing with pre-existing conditions (e.g., diabetes) whilst travelling	3.3
The recommended contents of a first aid kit	3.3
Travelling with a medical or first aid kit	3.2
Tropical diseases at their destination	2.9
Methods of water purification	2.9
The need for early diagnosis and treatment of malaria	2.8
Health issues of travelling with children	2.8
Altering dosages of medications when travelling through multiple time zones	2.7
Prevention and treatment of jet leg	2.6
Current disease outbreaks at their destination	2.5
Need for travel medical insurance	2.4
Health issues of travelling whilst pregnant	2.2
Risk and prevention of accidents whilst overseas	2.0
Risk and prevention of sexually transmitted diseases	2.0
How to obtain medical care whilst overseas	2.0
Prevention and treatment of acute mountain sickness	2.0
Safe alcohol and drug consumption whilst overseas	1.9
Issues regarding personal safety and crime prevention	1.9
Prevention and treatment of diving-related illnesses	1.7

Scale used: 1-Never advise, 2-Rarely advise, 3-Occasionally advise, 4-Frequently advise, 5-Always advise.

3.3. Future Practices

By rating their level of agreement or disagreement to standard statements with 5-point Likert scales, respondents gave their views regarding the current and future roles of Australian pharmacists in the area of travel health, potential barriers to service development and the training needs of pharmacists. Table 2 gives the respondents' average rating to each statement examining their views of travel health as an appropriate current and potential future role for Australian pharmacists in travel health. Table 2 also acts as the key for Figure 1, which summarises the percentage of the respondents who chose a particular rating for each statement.

Table 2. Average ratings for how frequently pharmacists agreed or disagreed to statements relating to the current or future roles of pharmacists in the area of travel health (n = 255).

Statement	Average Rating (Scale 1–5)
a. Travelers want pharmacists to offer travel health services	4.0
b. Pharmacists cannot offer adequate travel health services as they cannot administer vaccines	2.0
c. Pharmacists cannot offer adequate travel health services as they cannot supply S4 medications without prescription	3.0
d. Offering travel health services would cause antipathy with the medical profession	3.0
e. Travel health is not an appropriate role for pharmacists	2.0
f. The most appropriate role for pharmacists in travel health is to check the appropriateness of medications prescribed for the traveller	2.9
g. The pharmacist has a role advising travellers who would not normally visit a doctor before travelling on travel-related health issues	4.0
h. The pharmacist has a role advising travellers whether to seek medical advice before visiting certain destinations	4.0
i. The pharmacist can adequately advise the traveller on items to place in a first aid kit when travelling to remote destinations	4.4

Scale used: 1-strongly disagree, 2-disagree, 3-neutral (neither agree or disagree), 4-agree, 5-strongly agree.

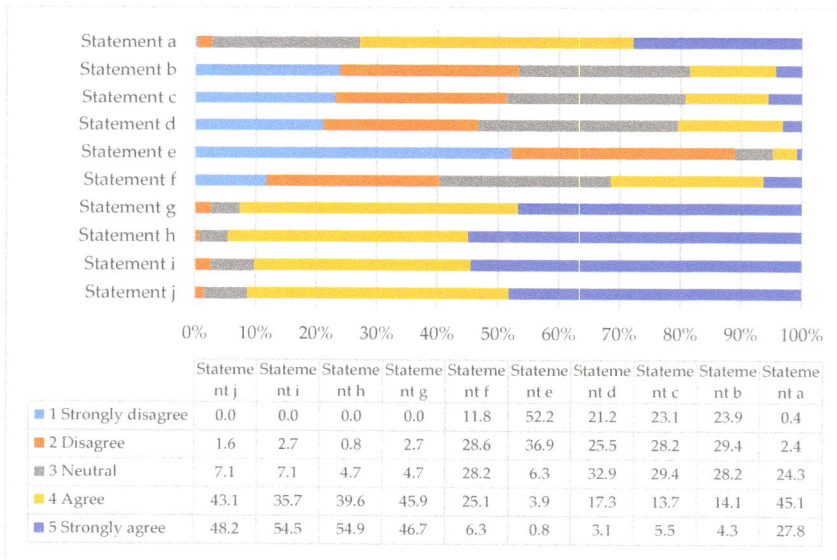

	Statement j	Statement i	Statement h	Statement g	Statement f	Statement e	Statement d	Statement c	Statement b	Statement a
1 Strongly disagree	0.0	0.0	0.0	0.0	11.8	52.2	21.2	23.1	23.9	0.4
2 Disagree	1.6	2.7	0.8	2.7	28.6	36.9	25.5	28.2	29.4	2.4
3 Neutral	7.1	7.1	4.7	4.7	28.2	6.3	32.9	29.4	28.2	24.3
4 Agree	43.1	35.7	39.6	45.9	25.1	3.9	17.3	13.7	14.1	45.1
5 Strongly agree	48.2	54.5	54.9	46.7	6.3	0.8	3.1	5.5	4.3	27.8

Figure 1. Percentage ratings of how frequently pharmacists agreed or disagreed to statements relating to the current or future roles of pharmacists in the area of travel health (n = 255).

Nearly 90% of respondents disagreed/strongly disagreed with statement *e* (average rating 2.0) thereby demonstrating that they consider travel health to be an appropriate role for pharmacists. In addition, because 72.9% of respondents agreed/strongly agreed with statement *a* (average rating

4.0), they also feel that travellers would support pharmacist-run travel health services. At the time of the survey it was uncommon for Australian pharmacies to offer vaccination services and they were and still are, unable to supply prescription only medications without a prescription from an appropriate prescriber. However, it appears that the respondents do not see this as a major barrier to travel health service development (53.3% and 51.3% of respondents disagreed/strongly disagreed with statements *b* and *c* respectively). In addition, although the safe dispensing and supply of medications is recognised as a core function of pharmacists in the healthcare system, responses suggest that respondents were divided as to whether this should be their only function in the area of travel health (40.4% disagreed/strongly disagreed to statement *f*, whereas, 31.4% agreed/strongly agreed and 28.2% appeared neutral). Responses suggest that they felt more strongly that suitable roles for pharmacists in travel health included giving travel health advice to travellers who would not normally obtain pre-travel advice from their doctor (92.6% agreed/strongly agreed with statement *g*), supplementing or reinforcing the advice given by other practitioners, advising on travel-related health issues that may not have been covered by their doctor (91.3% agreed/strongly agreed with statement *j*) and referring some travellers back to their doctor if they are visiting certain destinations, perhaps for vaccinations and antimalarials or other medications (94.5% agreed/strongly agreed with statement *h*). Finally, they agreed that pharmacists have a role in the supply of traveller's first aid kits and advising on their contents (90.2% agreed/strongly agreed with statement *i*).

Likewise, by rating their level of agreement/disagreement to standard statements using a 5-point Likert scale, respondents also gave their views relating to potential barriers to the development of pharmacist-run travel health services. Table 3 gives the respondents' average rating to each statement and also acts as the key for Figure 2 which summarises the percentage of the respondents who chose a particular rating for each statement.

Table 3. Average ratings for how frequently pharmacists agreed or disagreed to statements relating to potential barriers that may limit or slow the development of pharmacists' roles with regard to travel health (n = 255).

Statement	Average Rating (Scale 1–5)
a. The average community pharmacist would not have enough time to provide quality travel health services	3.4
b. My pharmacy has inadequate staffing levels to provide quality travel health services	3.0
c. Pharmacy assistants could advise travellers on travel-related health issues	3.0
d. Travelers do not want pharmacies to offer travel health services	2.0
e. Travel health services would not be profitable for pharmacies	3.0
f. I am not interested in providing travel health services	1.8
g. Pharmacists are inadequately trained to provide travel health services	3.0
h. The inability to supply S4 medications without prescription would make travel health services unviable from pharmacies	3.0
i. Perceived antipathy from other health professionals would stop me developing travel health services	2.3

Scale used: 1-strongly disagree, 2-disagree, 3-neutral (neither agree or disagree), 4-agree, 5-strongly agree.

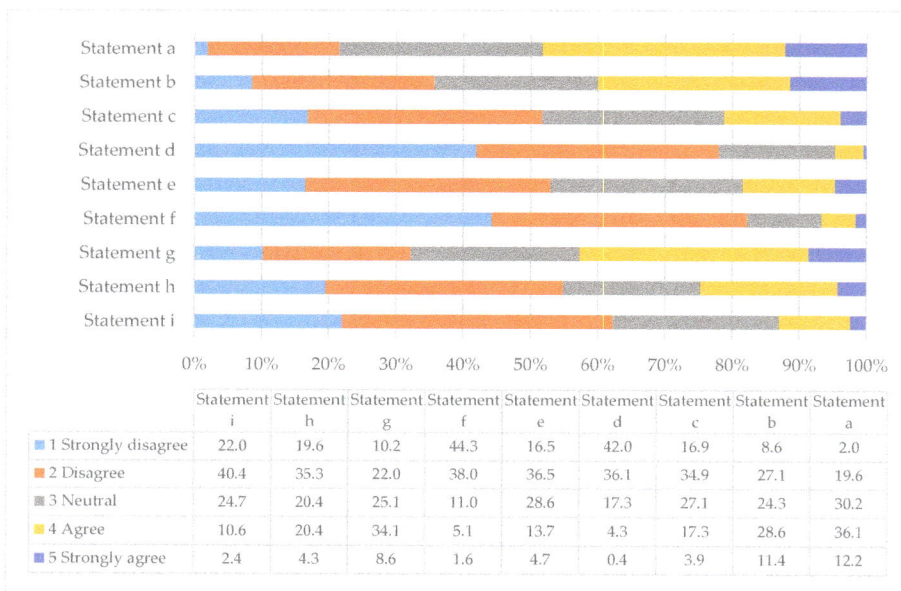

	Statement i	Statement h	Statement g	Statement f	Statement e	Statement d	Statement c	Statement b	Statement a
■ 1 Strongly disagree	22.0	19.6	10.2	44.3	16.5	42.0	16.9	8.6	2.0
■ 2 Disagree	40.4	35.3	22.0	38.0	36.5	36.1	34.9	27.1	19.6
▨ 3 Neutral	24.7	20.4	25.1	11.0	28.6	17.3	27.1	24.3	30.2
■ 4 Agree	10.6	20.4	34.1	5.1	13.7	4.3	17.3	28.6	36.1
■ 5 Strongly agree	2.4	4.3	8.6	1.6	4.7	0.4	3.9	11.4	12.2

Figure 2. Percentage ratings of how frequently pharmacists agreed or disagreed to statements relating to potential barriers that may limit of slow the development of pharmacists with regard to travel health (n = 255).

Although respondents were very interested in providing travel health services (82.3% disagreed/strongly disagreed with statement *f*), they did recognise both time and staffing to be potential barriers (48.3% and 40% agreed/strongly agreed to statements *a* and *b* respectively). However, responses were divided because 30.2% of respondents were also neutral to statement a (time) and 35.7% disagreed/strongly disagreed with statement *b* (staffing). One criticism of extended pharmacy services is that they are often undertaken by pharmacy assistants and not qualified pharmacists [20], however the respondents do not appear to view travel health as a potential role for pharmacy assistants (only 21.2% agreed/strongly agreed with statement *c*). Importantly, the respondents felt that travel health services from pharmacies could be profitable and, again, that the inability to supply prescription only medications without prescription would not adversely affect the viability of the service (53% and 54.9% of respondents disagreed/strongly disagreed with statements *e* and *h* respectively). It appears that respondents did not expect antipathy from the medical profession and, that even if this was the case, it would not prevent them from developing travel health services (62.4% disagreed/strongly disagreed with statement *i*).

Finally, although 68.2% (174/255) of the respondents provide some level of travel health service, the vast majority of respondents (96.9%, 247/255) had not received any formal travel health training. However, 42.7% of respondents did recognise that they require further training, if they wish to provide quality travel health services and the majority would wish that training to be accredited either by a pharmacy (41.6%, 106/255) or travel medicine (45.1%, 115/255) professional body. They would also prefer the training to be available either online (40%, 102/255) or using a combined on-line and block mode delivery method (52.5%, 134/255).

4. Discussion

At the time of the survey, few Australian pharmacies offered immunisation services and were and are currently, unable to supply antibiotics and antimalarial medications without a prescription.

However, a large number of respondents offered some form of travel health service and although most only responded to simple travel health enquires instigated by the traveller, a small number did offer comprehensive pre-travel health risk assessments for their clients. The travel health workload in all pharmacies appeared low. In contrast, although many of the reported international pharmacy-run travel health services appear to offer fully comprehensive services, supported with standard questionnaires and interview schedules to aid the assessment of travellers [13,15,17,21–23], their workload is also often low and comparable with that of this study. Kodkani et al. [18] also reported a variation in pharmacy travel health workload in Switzerland, with 8% of respondents giving frequent advice (more than 5 times per week) and 10% giving infrequent advice (less than 6 times per year). However, the majority of respondents (56%) in the Kodkani study only gave travel health advice to 2–3 clients per month. Likewise, Teodosio et al. [19] reported that 87.6% of Portuguese pharmacies in their study only advised up to 3 travellers per month.

Many of the respondents only discussed a limited range of health topics with their clients. However, the top ten topics that respondents most frequently discussed aligned with the recommended travel health counselling topics suggested by Spira [24]. These are also the topics of most interest to travellers, such as vaccinations and malaria chemoprophylaxis and issues relating to common travel-related conditions, such as Traveller's diarrhoea. However, the list also includes areas highlighted as key areas for pharmacist input, such as medication management and travel first aid kits. Topics rarely discussed with travellers included more specialised travel health situations, such as diving-related illness and acute mountain sickness. In addition, pharmacists rarely advised travellers about some relatively common travel health situations and issues, such as the risk or prevention of sexually transmitted diseases and accidents and how to obtain medical care overseas. There are many reasons why pharmacists do or do not counsel travellers on some topics with time limitations being a major factor, as is the perception by pharmacists as to their role, which may not extend to travel insurance, the prevention of accidents or diving and mountaineering-related issues. Other studies have examined the advice given to travellers by both doctors and pharmacists and some have found some deficiencies or omissions in the advice given [18,19,25,26]. For example, it was found that although high numbers of Swiss and German general practitioners (GPs) regularly gave travel health advice, many did not provide correct recommendations for vaccinations and malaria chemoprophylaxis for common tropical destinations [26]. Likewise, another study also found that some GPs also gave a limited range of pre-travel health advice and that, for example, over 50% of the GPs surveyed did not give travellers pre-travel advice on the risk and prevention of sexually transmitted diseases [27].

Travel health is a rapidly changing field and travel health providers must keep abreast of these changes, if they are to provide the most accurate and up to date information [28]. Some studies have examined the information resources used by other travel health providers such as GPs [26,28,29]. However, there appears to be little known about the information resources used by Australian pharmacists in the provision of travel health advice. It appears that the respondents tend to use more generic drug information resources and few specialist travel health information resources. However, the publications used are readily accessible, regularly up-dated and are fairly economical in price. Hatz et al. [26] found that Swiss GPs tend to prefer national resources and guides and Leggat and Seelan [28] also found that the Australian Immunisation Handbook was a commonly used resource by Australian GPs. Few of the respondents mentioned that they referred to peer reviewed journals for information, perhaps due to a lack of accessibility. This concurs with findings from Australian GPs by Leggat and Seelan [28].

The restrictions placed on Australian pharmacists offering vaccination services and to supply prescription only medications without a prescription could have been perceived as a barrier to travel health service development, however the results of this study show that this does not appear to be the case. In the UK and USA, the ability to offer vaccinations in pharmacies without prescription has been an important enabling factor for the development of pharmacy-run travel health services [9,13,30]. Therefore, as pharmacy immunisation services are now more common, it would be interesting to reinvestigate the views of Australian pharmacists about pharmacy-run travel health immunisation services in more detail. Inadequate staffing levels, time, lack of training and antipathy with other health professions are often listed as potential barriers to the development of extended services by pharmacists [31]. However, in this study antipathy from other health professionals did not appear to be a major concern for respondents and although staffing and time were reported as potential barriers, responses were also divided.

Finally, the fact that many respondents self-recognised the need for further training in order to deliver high quality travel health services is consistent with the findings of other studies [2,20] who also reported that the vast majority of respondents in their study (93.2%) had no training in travel medicine, however they did note that 77.9% did attempt to stay informed or be updated. Currently, there are no pharmacist-specific, accredited travel health training programs available for pharmacists in Australia. Therefore, this is an ideal opportunity for an Australian pharmacy professional body to work collaboratively with a peak travel health body, such as the International Society of Travel Medicine, in order develop a pharmacist-specific training program for Australian pharmacists to further progress the role of Australian pharmacists in this specialty area.

5. Conclusions

Findings from this study confirm that travel health is an appropriate role for Australian pharmacists and that their clients would seek travel health advice from pharmacies if offered. Therefore, there is consensus that expanding current practices from simple reactive services responding to travel-related enquiries to comprehensive pre-travel health risk assessments is an opportunity for future practice. Overcoming barriers of workload, time and the need for training will bring the Australian pharmacists into line with international practice and provide better outcomes for Australians travelling overseas.

Author Contributions: Conceptualization, I.M.H. and R.S.; Methodology, I.M.H.; Formal Analysis, I.M.H.; Investigation, I.M.H.; Data Curation, I.M.H.; Writing-Original Draft Preparation, I.M.H.; Writing-Review & Editing, I.M.H. and B.D.G.; Supervision, B.D.G., M.B. and R.S.; Project Administration, B.D.G.; Funding Acquisition, I.M.H.

Funding: This research was funded with a Faculty Allocated Internal Grant (FAIG) awarded by the Faculty of Medicine, Health and Molecular Sciences, James Cook University.

Conflicts of Interest: The authors declare no conflict of interest.

References

1. Glaesser, D.; Kester, J.; Paulose, H.; Alizadeh, A.; Valentin, B. Global travel patterns: an overview. *J. Travel. Med.* **2017**, *24*, 1–5. [CrossRef] [PubMed]
2. Houle, S.K.D. Pharmacy travel health services: current perspectives and future prospects. *Integr. Pharm. Res. Pract.* **2017**, *7*, 13–20. [CrossRef] [PubMed]
3. Van Herck, K.; Castelli, F.; Zuckerman, J.; Nothdurft, H.; Van Damme, P.; Dahlgren, A.L.; Gargalianos, P.; Lopéz-Vélez, R.; Overbosch, D.; Caumes, E.; et al. Knowledge, attitudes and practices in travel-related infectious disease: The European airport survey. *J. Travel. Med.* **2004**, *11*, 3–8. [CrossRef] [PubMed]
4. Wilder-Smith, A.; Khairullah, N.S.; Song, J.H.; Chen, C.Y.; Torresi, J. Travel health knowledge, attitudes and practices among Australasian travelers. *J. Travel. Med.* **2004**, *11*, 9–15. [CrossRef] [PubMed]
5. Toovey, S.; Jamieson, A.; Holloway, M. Travelers' knowledge, attitudes and practices on the prevention of infectious diseases: Results from a study at Johannesburg International Airport. *J. Travel. Med.* **2004**, *11*, 16–22. [CrossRef] [PubMed]
6. Hamer, D.H.; Connor, B.A. Travel health knowledge, attitudes and practices among United States travelers. *J. Travel. Med.* **2004**, *11*, 23–26. [CrossRef] [PubMed]
7. Namikawa, K.; Iida, T.; Ouchi, K.; Kimura, M. Knowledge, attitudes and practices of Japanese travelers on infectious disease risks and immunization uptake. *J. Travel. Med.* **2010**, *17*, 171–175. [CrossRef] [PubMed]
8. Goad, J.A. Travel medicine and the role of the pharmacist. *Adv. Pharm.* **2004**, *2*, 318–324.

9.   Hind, C.A.; Bond, C.M.; Lee, A.J.; Van Teijlingen, E.R. Needs assessment study for community pharmacy travel medicine services. *J. Travel. Med.* **2008**, *15*, 328–334. [CrossRef] [PubMed]

10.   Mason, P. What advice can pharmacists offer travellers to reduce their health risks? *Pharm. J.* **2004**, *273*, 651–656.

11.   Baker, L. The role of pharmacists in travel medicine in South Africa. *Pharmacy* **2018**, *6*, 68. [CrossRef] [PubMed]

12.   Evans, D. The impact of pharmacy based travel medicine with the evolution of pharmacy practice in the UK. *Pharmacy* **2018**, *6*, 64. [CrossRef] [PubMed]

13.   Hind, C.; Bond, C.; Lee, A.; van Teijlingen, E. Travel medicine services from a community pharmacy: Evaluation of a pilot service. *Pharm. J.* **2008**, *281*, 625.

14.   Bascom, C.S.; Rosenthal, M.M.; Houle, S.K. Are pharmacists ready for a greater role in travel health? An evaluation of the knowledge and confidence in providing travel health advice for pharmacists practicing in a community pharmacy chain in Alberta, Canada. *J. Travel. Med.* **2015**, *22*, 99–104. [CrossRef] [PubMed]

15.   Brennan, C. Pharmacist-run travel medicine clinic. *Ann. Pharmacother.* **2004**, *38*, 2168–2169. [CrossRef] [PubMed]

16.   Durham, M.J.; Goad, J.A.; Neinstein, L.S.; Lou, M. A comparison of pharmacist travel-health specialists' versus primary care providers' recommendations for travel-related medications, vaccinations, and patient compliance in a college health setting. *J. Travel. Med.* **2011**, *18*, 20–25. [CrossRef] [PubMed]

17.   Connelly, D. A pharmacist-led travel health clinic. *Pharm. J.* **2007**, *279*, 47.

18.   Kodkani, N.; Jenkins, J.M.; Hatz, C.F. Travel advice given by pharmacists. *J. Travel. Med.* **1999**, *6*, 87–92. [CrossRef] [PubMed]

19.   Teodosio, R.; Goncalves, L.; Imperatori, E.; Atouguia, J. Pharmacists and travel advice for tropics in Lisbon (Portugal). *J. Travel. Med.* **2006**, *13*, 281–287. [CrossRef] [PubMed]

20.   Hughes, C.M.; McCann, S. Perceived interprofessional barriers between community pharmacists and general practitioners. *Br. J. Gen. Pract.* **2003**, *53*, 600–606. [PubMed]

21.   Gatewood, S.B.S.; Stanley, D.D.; Goode, J.V.R. Implementation of a comprehensive pretravel health program in a supermarket chain pharmacy. *J. Am. Pharm. Assoc.* **2009**, *49*, 660–669. [CrossRef] [PubMed]

22.   Hess, K.M.; Dai, C.W.; Garner, B.; Law, A.V. Measuring outcomes of a pharmacist-run travel health clinic located in an independent community pharmacy. *J. Am. Pharm. Assoc.* **2010**, *50*, 174–180. [CrossRef] [PubMed]

23.   Goode, J.V.R.; Mott, D.A.; Stanley, D.D. Assessment of an immunization program in a supermarket chain pharmacy. *J. Am. Pharm. Assoc.* **2007**, *47*, 495–498. [CrossRef] [PubMed]

24.   Spira, A.M. Travel medicine I: Preparing the traveller. *Lancet* **2003**, *361*, 1368–1381. [CrossRef]

25.   Carroll, B.; Behrens, R.H.; Crichton, D. Primary health care needs for travel medicine training in Britain. *J. Travel. Med.* **1998**, *5*, 3–6. [CrossRef] [PubMed]

26.   Hatz, C.; Krause, E.; Grundmann, H. Travel advice: a study among Swiss and German general practitioners. *Trop. Med. Int. Health.* **1997**, *2*, 6–12. [CrossRef] [PubMed]

27.   Ropers, G.; Krause, G.; Tiemann, F.; Du Ry van Beest Holle, M.; Stark, K. Nationwide survey of the role of travel medicine in primary care in Germany. *J. Travel. Med.* **2004**, *11*, 287–294. [CrossRef] [PubMed]

28.   Leggat, P.A.; Seelan, S.T. Resources utilized by general practitioners for advising travelers from Australia. *J. Travel. Med.* **2003**, *10*, 15–18. [CrossRef] [PubMed]

29.   Leggat, P.A.; Heydon, J.L.; Menon, A. Resources used by general practitioners for advising travelers from New Zealand. *J. Travel. Med.* **2000**, *7*, 55–58. [CrossRef] [PubMed]

30.   Hind, C.; Downie, G. Vaccine administration in pharmacies—A Scottish success story. *Pharm. J.* **2006**, *277*, 134–136.

31.   Rosenthal, M.; Austin, Z.; Tsuyuki, R. Are pharmacists the ultimate barrier to pharmacy practice change? *Can. Pharm. J.* **2010**, *143*, 37–42. [CrossRef]

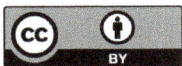

pharmacy

MDPI

Review

Pharmacy-Based Travel Health Services in the United States

Keri Hurley-Kim [1], Jeffery Goad [2], Sheila Seed [3] and Karl M. Hess [4,*]

1   Department of Pharmacy Practice, School of Pharmacy, West Coast University, Los Angeles, CA 90004, USA; khurley@westcoastuniversity.edu
2   Department of Pharmacy Practice, School of Pharmacy, Chapman University, Irvine, CA 92618, USA; goad@chapman.edu
3   Department of Pharmacy Practice, Massachusetts College of Pharmacy and Health Sciences University, Worcester, MA 01608, USA; sheila.seed@mcphs.edu
4   Department of Clinical and Administrative Sciences, School of Pharmacy and Health Sciences, Keck Graduate Institute, Claremont, CA 91711, USA
*   Correspondence: karl_hess@kgi.edu

Received: 30 October 2018; Accepted: 17 December 2018; Published: 27 December 2018

check for updates

Abstract: The aim of this paper is to review pharmacy laws and regulations, pharmacist training, clinic considerations, and patient care outcomes regarding pharmacy-based travel health services in the United States. Pharmacists and pharmacies in the United States are highly visible and accessible to the public, and have long been regarded as a source for immunization services. As international travel continues to increase and grow in popularity in this country, there is a pressing need for expanded access to preventative health services, including routine and travel vaccinations, as well as medications for prophylaxis or self-treatment of conditions that may be acquired overseas. In the United States, the scope of pharmacy practice continues to expand and incorporate these preventable health services to varying degrees on a state-by-state level. A literature review was undertaken to identify published articles on pharmacist- or pharmacy-based travel health services or care in the United States. The results of this paper show that pharmacists can help to increase access to and awareness of the need for these services to ensure that patients remain healthy while traveling abroad, and that they do not acquire a travel-related disease while on their trip. For those pharmacists interested in starting a travel health service, considerations should be made to ensure that they have the necessary training, education, and skill set in order to provide this specialty level of care, and that their practice setting is optimally designed to facilitate the service. While there is little published work available on pharmacy or pharmacist-provided travel health services in the United States, outcomes from published studies are positive, which further supports the role of the pharmacist in this setting.

Keywords: pharmacy law; education; training; vaccines; community pharmacy; ambulatory care

---

1. Background and Methods

In 2017, United States citizens made over 38 million visits to overseas international destinations, representing a 9% increase from the previous year, with this trend of increased travel expected to continue. According to the United States Department of Commerce, the most commonly reported purpose of travel was for vacation (55.8%), followed by visiting friends and relatives (26.7%) [1]. Regardless of the reason for travel, there are many risks involved when traveling to international destinations, from travelers' diarrhea to malaria to yellow fever. Unfortunately, 22 to 64% of travelers report some kind of health problem that might have otherwise been prevented with travel health services [2]. However, the main source for trip planning and preparation were the airlines (52.8%), followed by an online travel agency (33.1%), which may not be ideal sources for personalized health information, recommendations, and needed vaccines or medications [1].

The field of travel medicine can be broken down into pre- and post-travel health care. Pharmacists more commonly practice pre-travel health care or simply travel health, which focuses on preventable services prior to one's trip abroad. There is a growing need to expand access to and increase awareness of travel health services among the United States population. However, most estimates show that only about one-third to one-half of international travelers seek any form of travel health care prior to their departure from the United States [3,4]. Reasons for this include cost, accessibility, lack of awareness, and health disparities between specific U.S. populations [4–6]. Pharmacists can play a vital role in patient education and disease prevention related to international travel, due to their high visibility and accessibility to the public, particularly in community pharmacy settings, as well as their training. Pharmacists, depending upon state law, can often provide all necessary vaccines, medications, supplies, and in-depth patient counseling prior to their patient's departure. The purpose of this paper is therefore to highlight United States pharmacy laws and regulations, as well as pharmacist training, travel clinic considerations, and patient care outcomes from pharmacy-based travel health services. PubMed and the bibliography section of the Pharmacists Professional Group of the International Society of Travel Medicine were searched for published articles on pharmacist or pharmacy-based travel health services or care in the United States. Published articles from outside of the United States were not used for the purpose of this review. As a result, comparisons between the United States and other countries were not undertaken. Findings from these searches are provided below.

2. Main Findings

2.1. Pharmacists' Scope of Practice in Travel Health in the United States: Laws and Regulations

In the United States, the practice of pharmacy is regulated by individual states, thus there is sometimes significant variability in the care pharmacists are able to provide from one state to another. Despite this, pharmacists are highly trusted, visible to the public, and help to improve access to a variety of health care services [1–6]. Pharmacists continue to gain legal recognition as health care providers who can help support a health care system that is short on primary care physicians, nurses, and other providers. As such, the scope of pharmacists practice in certain areas, including travel health, is expanding.

Pharmacists in the United States have been providing immunizations and travel health care services for over 20 years [7,8]. The American Pharmacists Association (APhA) reports that more than 10,000 pharmacists have received specialized travel health training (B. Shah personal communication 18 November 2018). Historically, pharmacists have provided travel health services under protocols or collaborative practice agreements (CPA) with physicians in ambulatory care settings; however, several states and territories now allow for more independent practice [7–9].

The travel health services that pharmacists provide can be broken down into the provision of (1) counseling, (2) administering vaccines, (3) furnishing prescription medications, (4) ordering/interpreting laboratory tests, and (5) providing self-care medications and other supplies. Of 51 jurisdictions (U.S. States and Territories), 45 allow pharmacists to provide at least some level of travel health service beyond counseling and providing self-care medications and supplies (which are within the scope of practice for all pharmacists). This includes the administration of routine and travel health vaccines, self-treatment and secondary disease prevention medications, and prophylactic medications. Travel health services may also include ordering laboratory tests, such as titers, to assess immunity to vaccine-preventable diseases as well as G6PD deficiency testing [9].

Pharmacists in 15 jurisdictions can administer all routine vaccines independently. In 30 jurisdictions, a CPA or prescription is required. Pharmacists in eight jurisdictions can administer all travel-related vaccines independently, while a CPA or prescription is required in 36 jurisdictions. Pharmacists in 25 and 19 of the jurisdictions can furnish prescription medications and order laboratory tests under a CPA, respectively. There are also specific travel health training requirements in eight states (Alaska, Arkansas, California, Florida, New Mexico, Oregon, Rhode Island, and South Carolina) [9].

2.2. Notable Examples

In New Mexico, pharmacists can provide all aspects of care (administering vaccines, furnishing medications, and ordering laboratory tests) independently without collaborating with a physician. In California, pharmacists can independently provide routine immunizations and travel-related prescription medications that do not require a diagnosis, which includes chemoprophylaxis and self-treatment of travel-related conditions. A CPA, however, is still required in order to administer travel vaccines in this state. In Hawaii, pharmacists can independently administer all immunizations, including those for travel, but requires a CPA in order to furnish travel-related prescription medications. Pharmacists in these three states can also independently order laboratory tests. Finally, new laws and/or regulations are pending or were recently passed in at least six jurisdictions that will expand travel health scope of practice for pharmacists if enacted into law. Interestingly, pharmacy technicians in Idaho can now administer routine vaccines to patients, which may help facilitate pharmacist-provided patient care services in this state [9].

2.3. Pharmacist Training

The discipline of travel health involves a comprehensive knowledge and resource base, including infectious diseases, epidemiology, environmental, geographic, and consular matters related to travelers' health and safety [10]. Since this field is unique, dynamic, and a rapidly growing area of practice for pharmacists, it is important to maintain a high standard of practice. The following section outlines the educational and training requirements for pharmacists wanting to provide travel health services in the United States.

Providing comprehensive travel health services involves determining patients' specific travel health needs, providing immunizations, furnishing necessary medications, and counseling patients on health and safety risks specific to their destination and itinerary. Pharmacists in the United States interested in providing travel health services are encouraged to first complete a comprehensive immunization training program, such as the APhA Pharmacy-based Immunization Delivery Certificate Training Program (https://www.pharmacist.com/pharmacy-based-immunization-delivery) [11]. This program is comprised of a self-study and live training seminar offering 20 h continuing education. Although a general immunization-training program such as this one does not address specific travel-related vaccines in detail, it does provide a very robust and strong foundation of knowledge, practices, decision-making skills, regulations, and techniques related to immunization delivery that is necessary in patient care and travel health.

The successful completion of the APhA Pharmacy-Based Immunization Delivery Training program and being an authorized provider of immunizations in their state is a prerequisite to enroll in the APhA Advanced Competency Training Pharmacy-Based Travel Health Services program, which helps provide a solid foundation on which to build a travel health practice. This program offers 10 h of continuing education, and includes self-study and live seminar components that will prepare pharmacists to evaluate travel itineraries; assess health and safety risks based on travelers' destinations, reasons for travel, and medical history; and create and communicate a plan for patients to receive the necessary medications, immunizations, counseling, and non-prescription medications and supplies for their trip (https://www.pharmacist.com/pharmacy-based-travel-health-services) [12].

The gold standard in the scope of travel health knowledge is the "Body of Knowledge" developed by the International Society of Travel Medicine (ISTM). This "Body of Knowledge" serves as the basis for the Certificate of Knowledge examination that is available through the ISTM for all travel health professionals. Those who successfully complete the exam are awarded the Certificate in Travel Health (CTH) by the ISTM, which must be renewed every 10 years by continuous professional development or retesting. The CTH is one of few credentials offered across health professions and is recognized internationally (http://www.istm.org/bodyofknowledge) [13].

2.4. Resources

Once initial training is complete, pharmacists should maintain a comprehensive knowledge base of travel-related issues, in order to be prepared for any itinerary that may come their way. A well-informed travel health provider must have the appropriate resources to remain up-to-date on information, such as disease outbreaks, changes in country entry requirements, and vaccine recommendations [10]. The U.S. Centers for Disease Control and Prevention (CDC) maintains a list of Travel Medicine resources (https://wwwnc.cdc.gov/travel/page/travel-medicine-references) [14]. Additional travel health clinic considerations and logistics can be found in Table 1.

Table 1. Travel health clinic considerations and logistics [15,16].

Components	Comments
Patient education material	• Printed or electronic (must be current). • Patient-and itinerary-specific. • U.S. Centers for Disease Control and Prevention (CDC) and commercial sources have patient handouts.
Immunization	• With the exception of yellow fever vaccine, most immunizations are available to order through pharmacy wholesalers or other vaccine distributors. • Yellow fever vaccine is supplied directly by the manufacturer, and may only be ordered by facilities associated with an official yellow fever vaccine provider. • As with basic immunization services, it is important that all necessary supplies and equipment for administration are available and easily accessible. Close attention should be paid to the storage requirements of all vaccines. See the CDC's recommendation for proper storage and handling of all vaccines. (http://www.cdc.gov/vaccines/hcp/admin/storage/toolkit/index.html).

Provision of prescription medications	• Furnishing, prescribing, initiating, and ordering medications (term varies by state)
	• Medications recommended for international travel that the pharmacists may furnish or provide generally fall into two categories:
	  ○ self-treatment
	  ○ chemoprophylaxis.
	• The CDC Yellow Book details all drugs and conditions that fall into these categories.
	• Many travel health practices opt to use pre-populated checklist-type prescription forms, as the regimens for common travel related medications are standard. This may help to increase efficiency, consistency, and potentially reduce furnishing errors.
	• All furnishing pharmacists in need to obtain an individual National Provider Identification (NPI).

Laboratory tests	• State law dictates how or if pharmacists can order tests.
	• Antibody titers:
	  ○ Hepatitis A and B
	  ○ Varicella Zoster Virus (VZV)
	  ○ Measles, Mumps, and Rubella (MMR)
	  ○ Rabies
	• Glucose-6 Phosphate Dehydrogenase (G6PD) deficiency for primaquine and tafenoquine.

Table 1. *Cont.*

Components	Comments
Supplies	• Best to stock an adequate supply for sale, but can create patient handouts of supplies to obtain elsewhere. • Over-the-counter supplies. • Non-medication supplies.
Workflow	• Perform the risk assessment based on the patient's travel health history. • Prepare patient specific education documents and recommendations. • Provide the travel consultation. • Provide appropriate immunizations and documentation.
Staffing	• Marketing, patient scheduling and reminders, and vaccine/prescription input and billing can be delegated to a pharmacy technician, clerk, or intern pharmacist (i.e., a student pharmacist in training). • In an ambulatory care setting, nurses may also be used to perform clerical responsibilities and administer vaccinations. • A student pharmacist may also assist in the preparation of the consultation documents and recommendations, and preparation and administration of vaccinations if appropriately trained and supervised.
Space	• The space used for existing services, such as routine immunizations, is usually appropriate for providing travel health services. • A private clinic room is ideal, but not required, as patients may feel more comfortable discussing medical history and receiving immunizations in an enclosed area.
Scheduling of Patients	• Appointment (preferred), but can do walk-in. Schedule for a minimum of 30 minutes, depending upon the complexity of the visit. Ask patients to make appointments four to six weeks before departure. • Focused travel clinic visits rather than integrating with other services. • Consider group consults for families traveling together or groups with the same itinerary.
Documentation	• Documentation can be print or electronic—states that require immunization registry documentation will need electronic transmission. • A patient progress note that fully documents the clinical assessment and travel medication plan. • A patient medication record for each medication provided to the patient by the pharmacist. • Documentation of the administration of vaccines (vaccine name, lot number, expiration date, anatomical site vaccine administered, initials of pharmacist, date vaccine given, date of Vaccine Information Statement (VIS) • Documentation of yellow fever vaccination on the International Certificate of Vaccination or Prophylaxis (ICV-P) form with associated official stamp from the state health department when yellow fever vaccine is administered. • Documenting refrigerator and freezer temperatures at least twice a day following CDC recommendations. This is also a requirement of being a yellow fever vaccine provider.

2.5. Pharmacist and Physician Partnership for Travel Health Clinic Protocols

State laws may require the use of a standing order, protocol, or CPA in order to administer routine and travel-related vaccines. According to the APhA Immunization Certificate Training Program, items that should be included for any vaccine protocol include:

1. Statement of physician authorization for the pharmacist to administer vaccines
2. Qualifications of person(s) administering vaccines
3. Vaccine(s) covered in the standing order/protocol
4. Policies
5. Screening patients for indications and contraindications
6. Information to provide to patients (e.g., VIS)
7. How to administer vaccine (e.g., dose, route, anatomic location)
8. Documentation requirements
9. Communication to physician and reporting requirements
10. Emergency procedures (e.g., use of epinephrine for allergic reactions) including specific protocol

Please note that only physicians can apply to become yellow fever vaccine stamp holders, but they can designate other appropriately licensed individuals at designated yellow fever vaccine centers (http://wwwnc.cdc.gov/travel/yellow-fever-vaccination-clinics/search) to administer the yellow fever vaccine and sign the international certificate of vaccination (ICV-P) [17]. Both the physician and pharmacist need to complete the appropriate yellow fever application and submit any additional documentation for certification as required by state law.

A travel clinic protocol would, in addition to the above for vaccination, have provisions for ordering of prescription medications and ordering laboratory tests, as well as other provisions for operation (see Table 1). It is critical for pharmacists to understand that a travel immunization clinic is not a travel health clinic, and only a comprehensive travel health clinic approach that includes consultation, medications, and immunizations should be undertaken. In California, a joint statement from the state professional organizations established the standard for what a travel health clinic should provide [18]. California has a unique practice model among other states, in that pharmacists have specific authority in the law to furnish (same outcome as "prescribe") prescription medications without a CPA, or order from a physician for international travelers, while non-routine vaccines (e.g., yellow fever, typhoid, cholera, and Japanese encephalitis) still require a CPA [19].

3. Outcomes of Pharmacist-Provided Care in Travel Health

More than 300,000 pharmacists have been trained to immunize in the United States [20]. Furthermore, pharmacists in all fifty states and territories are able to provide immunizations with varying degrees of restrictions, dependent upon individual regulations [9,21]. Pharmacists have been increasingly involved with providing direct patient care services that depart from the traditional dispensing role, and providing travel health services is one such activity.

In the literature, there are a few descriptive examples of pharmacist-provided care in travel health in a variety of settings, such as supermarket chain pharmacies, independent community pharmacies, telepharmacy services, multidisciplinary outpatient clinics, and student health centers [22–25]. Travel health care should include comprehensive patient consultations, and include information on disease prevention and immunizations, malaria prophylaxis, travelers' diarrhea, insect protection, and safe food/water precautions as mentioned in the previous section [7,22–24]. Depending upon the type of population that the clinic serves, more specialty services could include high altitude expeditions, wilderness survival, diving, or other forms of adventure travel.

There are limited studies in the literature that have evaluated health outcomes in pharmacist-run travel clinics in the United States. Hess et al. evaluated over 250 patients' acceptance of pharmacist-made recommendations for vaccines and medications at an independent community pharmacy, with an 84.7% favorable patient response and a 96% patient satisfaction rate with the appointment. The study authors also showed that there was a statistically significant increase in patient knowledge of travel-related issues (medication use, adverse effects of medications, how to use insect repellents and insecticides, and how to safely consume food and water) following patient consultation. Patient satisfaction with the service also correlated with patient acceptance of pharmacist-made recommendations. This paper also documented what is believed to be the first travel health clinic located in an independent community pharmacy in the United States run solely by community pharmacists. Details on travel health clinic operations and logistics are also provided for those interested in starting up a similar service [23].

Tran et al. evaluated over 350 patients at a supermarket pharmacy. This study evaluated health outcomes, acceptance of pharmacists' travel health recommendations, and patient satisfaction. Patients overwhelming accepted pharmacists' recommendations for immunizations (82%–100%). Non-pharmacologic recommendations made by the pharmacist were highly accepted, at a rate of approximately 90% with regards to drinking bottled water, safe food recommendations, and the importance of washing hands. A reported 20% of patients experienced travelers' diarrhea while traveling; however, those that experienced diarrhea and used the medications recommended by the pharmacist saw their symptoms alleviated. Approximately 79% obtained information on the prevention of malaria and insect protection. More than 90% reported that they took the medications as directed, and none contracted malaria while traveling [26]. Both Hess et al. and Tran et al. reported high patient satisfaction rates (96% and 94%, respectively) with a pharmacist-run travel health clinic [23,26].

Durham et al. compared recommendations between trained pharmacists at a pharmacist-run travel clinic in a university student health clinic versus primary care providers (PCP) without specialized training. Of the 513 travelers reviewed, pharmacists were more likely to follow evidence-based guidelines in regards to prescribing antibiotics for travelers' diarrhea when indicated (96% versus 50%), prescribing appropriate antimalarial medications (98% versus 81%), and ordering more vaccines for patients (mean 2.77 versus 2.31). Patients were also more likely to fill antibiotic prescriptions from the pharmacists-led clinic than from prescriptions written by their PCP (75% versus 63%) [25].

These studies show high patient satisfaction rates with pharmacist-provided travel health services, including both pharmacologic and non-pharmacologic recommendations with promising health outcomes (see Table 2 for full details). Despite these high satisfaction rates, some patients refused the pharmacist's recommendation for various vaccines. Patient acceptance rates in Tran et al. ranged from 10% (for Japanese encephalitis) to 100% (for yellow fever) for travel-related vaccines, but routine vaccine acceptance rates ranged from 0% to 31% [26]. Hess et al. had similar acceptance rates of travel-related vaccines, ranging from 67% (for polio) to 97% (for yellow fever). Patients cited a self-perceived low risk of contracting illnesses, or were only focused on the travel-related vaccines, such as yellow fever or typhoid, and not on routine illnesses like influenza or measles, mumps, and rubella [23]. Durham et al. demonstrated that pharmacists with specialty training and CTH credentials were able to provide expert care for their patients in regards to travel health [25]. All studies demonstrated that pharmacists are integral in educating patients on how to maintain their health while traveling abroad. In an effort to decrease refusal rates and increase immunization rates, pharmacists need to be more effective in informing patients on the risks of contracting vaccine-preventable travel related infectious diseases during the pre-travel visit. More research on the impact of such education and health outcomes for patients traveling is needed.

Table 2. Outcomes from pharmacist-based travel health services.

Authors	Hess et al. [23]	Durham et al. [25]	Tran et al. [26]
Methods	Retrospective database review of patient records and prospective patient satisfaction survey (4-point Likert scale) of patients seen at a pharmacist-run travel health clinic in an independent pharmacy.	Retrospective chart review comparing patients seen by a clinical pharmacist in a pharmacist-run travel clinic or a primary care provider (PCP) for international travel at a student health center at a university.	Retrospective cross-sectional study conducted in supermarket pharmacy. Telephone interview (75-question survey) for those patients that received a travel consultation.
Number of Eligible Subjects/Completed Study	283/82	513/172 (PCP) and 341 (Pharmacist)	356/103
Demographics	Database review: Average age: 47 years Female: 59% Survey: Average age: 52 years Female: 69% Completed college: 39%	Average age (18-25 years): 74% Females: 64%	Average age: 44 years Male: 47% Completed college: 75%
Objectives	Evaluate effectiveness of a pharmacist-run travel clinic through analysis of patient acceptance and refusal rates of recommendations, changes in understanding of travel-related issues and patient satisfaction with services. Explore factors that influence recommendations made with the patient's understanding of travel-related issues and patient satisfaction.	Compare and assess travel-related vaccine and medication recommendations between primary care providers and clinical pharmacists, with a specialty in pre-travel health. Compare compliance of medications and vaccinations recommended in each group.	Evaluate health outcomes and acceptance rates of travel health recommendations made by a pharmacist, and assess patient satisfaction rates with travel health-related services.

Table 2. *Cont.*

Results

Acceptance of pharmacist recommended vaccines/medications:

Total acceptance rate: 85%
- Antimalarials: 94%
- Yellow fever: 97%
- Polio: 66%
- Meningococcal: 71%
- Typhoid: 77%
- Hepatitis A: 79%

Reasons for refusal:
- Perceived low-risk of illness: 52%
- Only wanted yellow fever vaccine: 14%
- Cost: 14%
- Do not like receiving vaccines or taking medications: 7%
- Not confident in recommendation made: 3%
- Concerned about possible adverse effects: 3%

Changes in patient understanding: Before and after (mean, *p*-value):
- How to use travel meds correctly: 2.51 vs. 3.82, $p < 0.05$
- Possible side effects of travel medications: 2.4 vs. 3.75, $p < 0.05$
- How to use insect repellents correctly: 2.95 vs. 3.73, $p < 0.05$
- How to safely consume food and water: 3.22 vs. 3.82, $p < 0.05$

Overall patient satisfaction*: 3.73 (mean)

Pharmacist vs. PCP

Ordered antibiotics when indicated: 96% vs. 50%, $p < 0.0001$

Received antibiotics: 74.62% vs. 62.96%, $p = 0.0359$

Ordered antimalarial when indicated: 97.78% vs. 81.02%, $p < 0.001$

Received antimalarials: 81.48% vs. 86.36%, $p = 0.2657$

Ordered vaccines when indicated (mean number of vaccines): 2.78 vs. 2.06, $p < 0.0001$

Received vaccines (mean number of vaccines): 2.38 vs. 1.95, $p = 0.0039$

Acceptance of immunization recommendations:
- Hepatitis A: 67%
- Hepatitis B: 19%
- Influenza: 13%
- Japanese encephalitis: 10%
- Meningococcal: 18%
- Measles, mumps, rubella: 31%
- Polio: 79%
- Typhoid: 82%
- Yellow fever: 100%

Accepting pharmacist travel health recommendations:
- Prevention of sunburn:
  ○ Applied sunscreen: 87%
- Prevention of travelers' diarrhea:
  ○ Washed hands: 89%
  ○ Drank bottled water: 89%
  ○ Ate well-cooked food: 82%
- Insect protection:
  ○ Applied insect repellent: 61%
  ○ Wore protective clothing: 61%
  ○ Obtained antimalarial medications: 79% (of which 92% completed therapy)
- Prevention of altitude sickness:
  ○ Ascended slowly: 75%
  ○ Ate high-carbohydrate diet: 17%

Health Outcomes:
- 20% reported adverse effects with immunizations
- 5% reported a sunburn during their trip
- 20% reported travelers' diarrhea during trip
- 26% reported mosquito bites during their trip
- 0% reported contracting malaria
- 0% reported altitude sickness

Overall patient satisfaction**: 4.75 (mean)

Table 2. *Cont.*

| Limitations | Low response rate (29%), potential for recall bias since the survey was completed up to 1 year after clinic visit. | Not generalizable to general population, since the study only consisted of college-aged students. Could not control for differences in postgraduate training of the PCP's. | Low response rate (29%), the survey was delivered by telephone, and did not include questions on why the patient did not accept or follow the recommendations completely during travel. |

PCP: Primary Care Provider; * 4-point Likert scale; ** 5-point Likert scale.

4. Conclusions

The main limitation of this review is the lack of previously published literature that describes and assesses pharmacy- and pharmacist-provided travel health services in the United States. However, this paper adds to existing literature and provides an overview of the status of travel health care in the United States, including current U.S. pharmacy laws and regulations. Furthermore, practical considerations to incorporate such services has been provided to help further expand patient access to this needed service. This, in turn, may help to increase awareness of travel-related disease risks among the traveling public, and help to drive utilization of travel health care into the pharmacy setting.

Author Contributions: All authors contributed equally to this paper.

Funding: This research received no external funding.

Conflicts of Interest: The authors declare no conflict of interest. Karl Hess, PharmD declares he is a speaker for Merck & Co. Jeff Goad, Pharm.D., MPH declares he is a speaker for Merck & Co, an advisor to PaxVax and Shoreland Travax and served on advisory boards for Sanofi Pasteur, GSK and Pfizer.

References

1. ITA Office of Travel and Tourism Industries. US Outbound Travel by World Regions. Available online: http://tinet.ita.doc.gov/outreachpages/outbound.general_information.outbound_overview.asp (accessed on 13 June 2018).

2. Steffen, R. Epidemiology: Morbidity and Mortality in Travelers. In *Travel Medicine*; Keystone, J.S., Ed.; Elsevier: London, UK, 2004; pp. 5–12.

3. LaRocque, R.C.; Rao, S.R.; Tsibris, A.; Lawton, T.; Anita Barry, M.; Marano, N.; Brunette, G.; Yanni, E.; Ryan, E.T. Pre-travel health advice-seeking behavior among US international travelers departing from Boston Logan International Airport. *J. Travel Med.* **2010**, *17*, 387–391. [CrossRef] [PubMed]

4. Hamer, D.H.; Conner, B.A. Travel health knowledge, attitudes and practices among United States travelers. *J. Travel Med.* **2004**, *11*, 23–26. [CrossRef] [PubMed]

5. Leonard, L.; Van Landingham, M. Adherence to travel health guidelines: The experience of Nigerian immigrants in Houston, Texas. *J. Immigr. Health* **2001**, *3*, 31–45. [CrossRef] [PubMed]

6. Angell, S.Y.; Cetron, M.S. Health disparities among travelers visiting friends and relatives abroad. *Ann. Intern. Med.* **2005**, *142*, 67–72. [CrossRef] [PubMed]

7. Seed, S.M.; Spooner, L.M.; O'Connor, K.; Abraham, G.M. A Multidisciplinary approach in travel medicine: The pharmacist perspective. *J. Travel Med.* **2011**, *18*, 352–354. [CrossRef] [PubMed]

8. Jackson, A.B.; Humphries, T.L.; Nelson, K.M.; Helling, D.K. Clinical pharmacy travel medicine services: A new frontier. *Ann. Pharmacother.* **2004**, *38*, 2160–2165. [CrossRef] [PubMed]

9. Hurley-Kim, K.; Snead, R.; Hess, K.M. Pharmacists' scope of practice in travel health: A review of state laws and regulations. *J. Am. Pharm. Assoc.* **2018**, *58*, 163–167. [CrossRef] [PubMed]

10. Hill, D.R.; Ericsson, C.D.; Pearson, R.D.; Keystone, J.S.; Freedman, D.O.; Kozarsky, P.E.; DuPont, H.L.; Bia, F.J.; Fischer, P.R.; Ryan, E.T. The practice of travel medicine: Guidelines by the Infectious Diseases Society of America. *Clin. Infect. Dis.* **2006**, *43*, 1499–1539. [CrossRef] [PubMed]

11. American Pharmacists Association. Pharmacy Based Immunization Delivery. Available online: https://www.pharmacist.com/pharmacy-based-immunization-delivery (accessed on 25 October 2018).

12. American Pharmacists Association. Pharmacy Based Travel Health Services. Available online: https://www.pharmacist.com/pharmacy-based-travel-health-services (accessed on 25 October 2018).

13. International Society of Travel Medicine. ISTM Certificate of Knowledge. Available online: http://www.istm.org/bodyofknowledge (accessed on 25 October 2018).

14. Centers for Disease Control and Prevention. Travel Medicine References: Books, Journals Articles, and Websites. Available online: https://wwwnc.cdc.gov/travel/page/travel-medicine-references (accessed on 25 October 2018).

15. Gregorian, T.; Bach, A.; Hess, K.; Goad, J.; Mirzaian, E. Implementing Pharmacy-Based Travel Health Services: Insight and Guidance from Frontline Practitioners. *Calif. Pharm. J.* **2017**, *LXIV*, 23–29.

16. Centers for Disease Control and Prevention. Vaccine Storage and Handling Toolkit. Available online: http://www.cdc.gov/vaccines/hcp/admin/storage/toolkit/index.html (accessed on 25 October 2018).

17. Centers for Disease Control and Prevention. Available online: http://wwwnc.cdc.gov/travel/yellow-fever-vaccination-clinics/search (accessed on 25 October 2018).

18. Goad, J.; Dudas, V.; Gregorian, T.; McCabe, J.; Hess, K.; Soleimanpou, S. Practice of Travel Health for Pharmacists. Joint California Pharmacist Association and California Society of Health-Systems Pharmacists Sub-Commit-Tee on SB493 Travel Medicine Provision. June 2016. Available online: https://tinyurl.com/travelhealthCA (accessed on 1 December 2018).

19. Pharmacists Furnishing Travel Medications, Division 17 of Title 16 of the California Code of Regulations. Available online: https://www.pharmacy.ca.gov/laws_regs/1746_5_oa.pdf (accessed on 1 December 2018).

20. American Pharmacists Association (APhA). APhA Honors 2018 Immunization Champions. Available online: https://www.pharmacist.com/article/apha-honors-2018-immunization-champions (accessed on 30 May 2018).

21. Hogue, M.D.; Grabenstein, J.D.; Foster, S.L.; Rotholz, M.C. Pharmacist involvement with immunizations: A decade of professional advancement. *J. Am. Pharm. Asscoc.* **2006**, *46*, 168–182. [CrossRef]

22. Gatewood, S.B.; Stanley, D.D.; Goode, J.V. Implementation of a comprehensive pretravel health program in a supermarket chain pharmacy. *J. Am. Pharm. Assoc.* **2009**, *49*, 660–669. [CrossRef] [PubMed]

23. Hess, K.M.; Dai, C.W.; Garner, B.; Law, A.V. Measuring Outcomes of a Pharmacist-Run Travel Health Clinic Located Within an Independent Community Pharmacy. *J. Am. Pharm. Assoc* **2010**, *50*, 174–180. [CrossRef] [PubMed]

24. Helling, D.K.; Nelson, K.M.; Ramirez, J.E.; Humphries, T.L. Kaiser Permanente Colorado region pharmacy department: Innovative leader in pharmacy practice. *J. Am. Pharm. Assoc.* **2006**, *46*, 67–76. [CrossRef]

25. Durham, M.J.; Goad, J.A.; Neinstien, L.S.; Lou, M. A comparison of pharmacist travel-health specialists' versus primary care providers' recommendations for travel-related medications, vaccination, and patient compliance in a college health setting. *J. Travel Med.* **2011**, *18*, 20–25. [CrossRef] [PubMed]

26. Tran, D.; Gatewood, S.; Moczygemba, L.R.; Stanley, D.D.; Goode, J.V. Evaluating health outcomes following a pharmacist-provided comprehensive pretravel health clinic in a supermarket pharmacy. *J. Am. Pharm. Assoc.* **2015**, *55*, 143–152. [CrossRef] [PubMed]

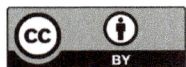

pharmacy

MDPI

Review

Multidisciplinary Collaboration between a Community Pharmacy and a Travel Clinic in a Swiss University Primary Care and Public Health Centre

Jérôme Berger [1,2,*], Marie-José Barbalat [1,3], Vanessa Pavón Clément [1,3], Blaise Genton [3,4,5] and Olivier Bugnon [1,2]

[1] Community Pharmacy Centre, Department of Ambulatory Care and Community Medicine, University of Lausanne, CH-1011 Lausanne, Switzerland; marie-jose.barbalat@hospvd.ch (M.-J.B.); vanessa.pavon-clement@hospvd.ch (V.P.C.); olivier.bugnon@hospvd.ch; (O.B.)
[2] Community Pharmacy Practice Research, School of pharmaceutical Sciences, University of Geneva/University of Lausanne, CH-1206 Genève, Switzerland
[3] Travel Clinic, Department of Ambulatory Care and Community Medicine, University of Lausanne, CH-1011 Lausanne, Switzerland; blaise.genton@chuv.ch
[4] Infectious Disease Service, University Hospital, CH-1011 Lausanne, Switzerland
[5] Swiss Tropical and Public Health Institute, CH-4051 Basel, Switzerland
* Correspondence: jerome.berger@hospvd.ch; Tel.: +41-21-314-78-55

Received: 7 November 2018; Accepted: 30 November 2018; Published: 5 December 2018

check for updates

Abstract: This review is a narrative description of a collaboration between a travel clinic and a community pharmacy centre within a university primary care and public health centre (Lausanne/Switzerland). Pharmacists and pharmacy technicians participate in this collaboration to provide (1). counselling and clinical activities with travellers (e.g., pre-travel consultations and advice to travellers), (2). clinical pharmacy expertise and medicine information services (e.g., selection of an appropriate antimalarial medication for a traveller to manage of drug-drug interactions), (3). technical and logistical activities related to medicines and vaccines (e.g., management of vaccine shortages and specially imported medicines and vaccines from foreign countries) and (4). educational activities (e.g., undergraduate pharmacy teaching and continuous education to community pharmacists). Such a multidisciplinary collaboration should be encouraged as it enables us to address the evolution and challenges of travel medicine related to medication, such as growing vaccine shortages and an increasing number of chronic patients who travel. This review may be used as a model for the dissemination of such collaborative practices, to develop future advanced teaching and training activities, to provide a framework for research related to travel and medicines and to participate in the evaluation of vaccination practices by community pharmacists.

Keywords: travel medicine; pharmacy; community; travel; practice; vaccination; Switzerland; multidisciplinary collaboration

---

1. Introduction

The Department of Ambulatory Care and Community Medicine of Lausanne (in the French-speaking part of Switzerland) is a university primary care and public health centre with health care workers that include general practitioners, nurse practitioners, and community pharmacists. Almost 600 people work in this centre, including 145 physicians and 172 other health care professionals (such as nurses and community pharmacists). Next to its community pharmacy centre (which includes a community pharmacy as well as a research unit), the centre hosts a travel clinic, where physicians, nurses, pharmacists and pharmacy technicians care for adult, geriatric and child travellers. The head of the community pharmacy centre is a professor of pharmacy practice and the head of the travel clinic is a professor of tropical and travel medicine. This academic setting facilitates the development of collaborative practice and of research and teaching activities.

The travel clinic is one of the two major centres in the French-speaking part of Switzerland. In 2017, the clinic administered 3900 yellow fever vaccines and performed more than 11,000 pre-travel consultations. The Swiss mandatory health insurance does not reimburse patients for pre-travel consultations. Hence, to ensure an affordable service, the aim of the travel clinic is to provide a standard pre-travel consultation in approximately 20 min. Post-travel consultations (e.g., for a traveller who is referred by the emergency department concerning a health problem after returning from a trip abroad) are also performed in the clinic. The characteristics of the travellers who are consulted in this travel clinic have already been described elsewhere [1]. In brief, the mean age of travellers is 32 years. Pre-travel consultations are sought approximately one month before departure (median of 29 days). Forty-six percent of travellers had at least one pre-existing medical condition (e.g., 9.4% reported a psychological or psychiatric problem, 1.8% a cancer and 0.4% an HIV infection). Most of them were travelling to Africa (46%), followed by Asia (35%) and Latin America (20%). Tourism (75%) and visits to friends and relatives (18%) were the main reported reasons to travel. At least one vaccine was administered to 99% of travellers [1].

The aim of this review is to present the multidisciplinary activities that occur within the travel clinic among physicians, nurses, community pharmacists and pharmacy technicians, as well as the educational activities of pharmacists related to travel medicine and vaccines.

2. Materials and Methods

To conduct this review, data were collected regarding the training of pharmacists involved in clinical activities with travellers, the activities and services of pharmacists and pharmacy-technicians related to the travel clinic and the educational activities of the pharmacy centre related to travel medicine and vaccines. Data assessment was based on the review of: 1. the 2017 annual report of the Department of Ambulatory Care and Community Medicine of Lausanne that summarizes clinical, research and educational activities; 2. the 2017 statistical directory of the Department of Ambulatory Care and Community Medicine of Lausanne that provides the main management indicators (e.g., number of patients, staff resources and budgets); 3. data extracted from custom-made software (DIAMM/G) that records the clinical activities in the travel clinic and 4. data extracted from custom-made administrative software (Allegro) used for human resources management by the Department of Ambulatory Care and Community Medicine of Lausanne. The findings are presented as a narrative description.

3. Results and Discussion

The main activities (summarized in Table 1) include counselling and clinical activities with travellers, providing clinical pharmacy expertise and medicines information services, technical and logistical activities related to medicines and vaccines and education activities.

Table 1. Main figures related to the activities of pharmacists and pharmacy-technicians within the travel clinic or related to travel medicine and vaccines (data from 2017).

Main Activities	Main Figures (From 1 January to 31 December 2017)
Counselling and clinical activities with travellers	<ul><li>303 pre-travel consultations managed by pharmacists</li><li>Approximately 3600 travellers supplied with medicines, sanitary materials or pharmacy kits by pharmacy technicians</li></ul>
Clinical pharmacy expertise and medicines information services	804 questions from the travel clinic managed by pharmacists
Technical and logistical activities related to medicines and vaccines	17 temperature excursion management activities in the travel clinic
Education Activities	<ul><li>8 h of undergraduate pharmacy teaching (travellers' counselling in the community pharmacy and immunization)</li><li>4 seminars (1–2 h) for community pharmacists (updates to vaccination schemes)</li><li>4 full days for pharmacy technicians (vaccination booklets and advice on vaccinations)</li><li>5 full days for pharmacists (immunization training, vaccination schemes and management of information)</li></ul>

3.1. Counselling and Clinical Activities with Travellers

Since 2009, pharmacists have been involved in the counselling and clinical activities of the travel clinic. As nurses and physicians consulting in the travel clinic, the pharmacists give advice according to travel purposes and patterns and the medical conditions of travellers, perform vaccinations (e.g., vaccinations for yellow fever, typhoid, rabies, and others), prescribe antimalarial medicines (for prophylaxis or stand-by emergency treatment) and collect blood samples for serology.

Currently, two pharmacists perform regular activities in the travel clinic. In 2017, they managed 137 and 166 pre-travel consultations, respectively. These pharmacists have been specifically trained to join the travel clinic. Their training was certified by a "Certificate in Travel Health" (International Society of Travel Medicine), a "Certificate of Achievement of Pharmacy-Based Immunization Delivery" (American Pharmacist Association) and a (in French) "Certificat de formation complémentaire FPH Vaccination et prélèvements sanguins (Foederatio Pharmaceutica Helvetiae)" [2]. The latter is a Swiss post-graduate training certificate that is mandatory for pharmacists who administer vaccines and it demonstrates skills in vaccination, injections and blood sample collection and processing techniques. In Switzerland, pharmacists who perform vaccinations must follow a mandatory training day every for two years to renew their "Certificat de formation complémentaire FPH Vaccination et prélèvements sanguins". In addition to this mandatory education, both pharmacists also completed continuing education on vaccines and travel medicine by participating in the monthly seminar held by the travel clinic and by attending the "Swiss Tropical and Public Health Institute - International Short Course on Travellers' Health", the (in French) "Congrès Suisse de Vaccination" and the (in French) "Journée Romande de Médecine des Voyages".

Under the supervision of pharmacists, pharmacy technicians take part in the travel clinic activities. The technicians charge the amounts that are linked to pre-travel consultations. This administrative task gives them the opportunity to complete the prevention and care advice for the travellers, mainly on the responsible use of antimalarial medicines (e.g., management of missed doses), safe sex, sun protection, mosquito bite prevention, water purification and treatment for motion sickness. If needed, technicians can supply travellers with medicines prescribed during the pre-travel consultations (e.g., antimalarials, antibiotics, preventive or acute treatment of altitude sickness) and they can deliver non-prescription medicines (e.g., antiemetics or antidiarrheals). Various items, such as sun protections, water filters, tablets for water disinfection, and mosquito nets or repellents, are actively promoted if needed. In 2017, pharmacy technicians delivered medicines, sanitary materials and/or pharmacy kits to approximately 3600 travellers after their pre-travel consultation at the travel clinic. Travellers are also free to buy medicines and other items in their usual community pharmacy.

3.2. Clinical Pharmacy Expertise and Medicines Information Services

In addition to the two pharmacists providing consultations in the travel clinic, other pharmacists also support the travel clinic activities. A medicines information service (MIS), run by pharmacists, is available from Monday to Saturday. The MIS offers a helpline related to medication management for health care professionals and patients and it manages the access to several medicine databases and to specific resources related to vaccines or travel medicine. The MIS also develops and updates practice recommendations and databases to promote the responsible use of medicines, such as antimalarials or vaccines. Such tools and databases include a drug-drug interaction database specifically dedicated to antimalarials, a database on temperature excursion management and several medicine comparison charts related to antimalarials, anti-infectives, vaccines and medications used in the prevention of deep vein thrombosis. The MIS also publishes patient information leaflets in French related to the use of anti-infectives that are not marketed in Switzerland but that may be prescribed by the travel clinic. Such medicines are imported from foreign countries (see below), and their packages do not include a patient leaflet in French. These medicines include diethylcarbamazine, niclosamid, praziquantel or primaquine. In addition, the MIS publishes patient information leaflets on travelling with medicines and supports the provision of certificates for carrying medicines (including narcotics).

In 2017, the MIS answered approximately 1800 phone requests, mainly from health care professionals within the primary care and public health centre. Among these, 804 questions were raised by the travel clinic. Questions from the travel clinic were mostly asked by nurses (81%), followed by physicians (12%). The majority (80%) concerned drug-drug interactions with antimalarials, either as chemoprophylaxis or as stand-by emergency treatment. Consultation with the MIS allows care providers to select the safest antimalarials, considering the individual medication plan of the travellers and according to their medical conditions (e.g., contraindications or allergies). The development and updates of internal tools and databases and the training of pharmacists mean that most of these 804 questions can be answered in a period that is compatible with pre-travel consultations: 79% of the questions were answered in less than 5 min and 17% in 6 to 15 min. One of the advantages of such a helpline is to allow clinicians to focus on the pre-travel consultation, while a pharmacist works in parallel to check for potential drug-drug interactions and looks for the best alternatives, if necessary, allowing the consultations to be shortened.

3.3. Technical and Logistical Activities Related to Medicines and Vaccines

In addition to consultation activities, the community pharmacy team ensures good provision and distribution of medicines and vaccines that are administered at the travel clinic or delivered to travellers. The supply chain of medicines and vaccines is ensured by the pharmacy, from orders to the stock management within the consulting rooms and fridges, including the proper disposal of unused medicines and vaccines. Such activity includes a continuous control by pharmacy technicians of the temperature of the cooling chamber and refrigerators used to stock vaccines in the travel clinic. In the case of an alarm (i.e., if the recorded temperature goes below 2 °C or above 8 °C), the MIS determines the action to take based on a database related to temperature excursion management. In 2017, the pharmacy managed 17 alarms in the travel clinic.

The pharmacy team also manages medicines and vaccine shortages, which are more and more frequent [3], in collaboration with physicians from the travel clinic. For example, in the case of a vaccine shortage, the pharmacy team gathers information on the currently available stock in the pharmacy and travel clinic, the recent number of injections of the vaccine, the probable next availability of the vaccine and the potential available alternatives (e.g., to continue vaccination schemes). Based on this information, a potential restricted administration of the vaccine during the shortage is discussed (e.g., which travellers should be vaccinated, with priority depending on their medical conditions and planned trips). This information is then disseminated within the travel clinic (e.g., the remaining stock of a vaccine may be taken out of the travel clinic to the pharmacy and delivered to health care professionals on request for administration to travellers who meet pre-established medical or travel conditions). In addition, a list of information and practice recommendations are made available to the pharmacy team to answer to other community pharmacies or physicians seeking for advice on the management of vaccine shortages.

Finally, importing special medicines and vaccines that are not marketed in Switzerland is performed by the pharmacy team for the travel clinic. Based on legal requirements, the pharmacy requests required import licenses from national health authorities (Swissmedic). In Switzerland, this is mandatory for vaccines imported from foreign countries [4]. In such cases, the pharmacy requests authorization to administer a foreign vaccine and authorizations linked to the import of every batch of a vaccine. Once all authorizations have been obtained, the pharmacy coordinates the importation process with a foreign wholesaler and Swiss customs. The entire process includes completing the requested forms (including clinical reasons to import a foreign vaccine, information on the pharmaceutical company, the clinicians who are responsible for administration of the vaccine and other information), paying the due taxes and ensuring full traceability of such imported vaccines (from information on the number of vaccines and batch numbers that have been received to the identities of the patients who have been administered injections). For example, 250 doses of typhoid-injectable vaccines were specially imported in five orders from France in 2017, because no such vaccine is marketed in Switzerland. These vaccines are indicated for patients in whom an oral live typhoid vaccine is contraindicated (e.g., in the case of drug-drug interactions, contraindications or too short of a delay prior to potential typhoid exposure).

3.4. Education Activities

The expertise gathered during the multidisciplinary activities at the travel clinic allows the pharmacists of the Department of Ambulatory Care and Community Medicine to teach other community pharmacists, pharmacy technicians and students about vaccines and travel medicine. For more than 10 years, master's students at the University of Geneva have been taught 4 h of education in the community pharmacy on counselling travellers (e.g., malaria prevention or travelling with medicines) and 4 h on immunization (e.g., vaccination schemes, vaccination booklets, advice on vaccinations in the community pharmacy). In the near future, injection and blood sample collection techniques will also be included in the master's programme. Indeed, pharmacists have been authorized to administer vaccines (e.g., influenza) in Switzerland for some years (depending on the canton). These new undergraduate courses will fulfil the revised national learning objectives for pharmacists, based on the Swiss Federal Act on Medical Professions [5].

In 2017, the pharmacy team offered continuous education sessions on vaccines and travel medicine to community pharmacists and pharmacy technicians in several locations throughout the French-speaking part of Switzerland. Four seminars (lasting 1 to 2 h) were conducted on updates to vaccination schemes for community pharmacists. Four full days of training were conducted for pharmacy technicians on the management of vaccination booklets (paper and electronic versions) and advice on vaccination in community. Finally, five full days (including case studies) of training were conducted for community pharmacists on immunizations, vaccination schemes and the management of information on sources on immunizations.

4. Conclusions

To the best of our knowledge, this report describes a unique example of a multidisciplinary collaboration between a university travel clinic and a university community pharmacy centre, at least in Switzerland. This report describes the benefits of a collaborative practice between pharmacists, pharmacy technicians, nurses and physicians in the activities of a travel clinic. As pharmacists and pharmacy technicians take part in the counselling and clinical activities with travellers, they gain knowledge and competence related to travel medicine and vaccines. Additionally, pharmacists and pharmacy technicians can bring their specific expertise and knowledge related to the responsible use of medicines to the travel clinic.

This effort goes beyond daily interactions between colleagues or completing the delivery of prescribed medicines and immunizations with responsible self-medication. This type of comprehensive collaborative practice is an advantage for travellers and for health professionals. Indeed, this practice supports the evolution of travel medicine and allows care providers to better face the challenges of travel medicine related to medications, such as growing vaccine shortages, an increasing number of chronic patients who travel and the increasing complexity of medicines administered while travelling abroad, such as self-administered injectables. As pharmacists are authorized to perform vaccinations in several countries and in most of the Swiss cantons, collaborations with travel clinics should be encouraged. The present review could serve as a model for the dissemination of such practices. The experience gained should form the basis for further teaching and training activities, including advanced training for pharmacists who are already authorized to perform vaccinations. In addition, this narrative may provide a framework for research related to travel, vaccines and medicines (e.g., evaluation of vaccination practices by community pharmacists or assessment of medication safety of chronic patients who travel).

Funding: This research received no external funding.

Acknowledgments: The authors thank C. Mialet for her assistance in collecting data related to the activity in the travel clinic.

Conflicts of Interest: The authors declare no conflicts of interest.

References

1. Dekkiche, S.; de Valliere, S.; D'Acremont, V.; Genton, B. Travel-related health risks in moderately and severely immunocompromised patients: A case-control study. *J. Travel Med.* **2016**, *23*. [CrossRef] [PubMed]
2. Foederatio Pharmaceutica Helvetiae. Formation Postgrade FPH—Vaccination et Prélèvements Sanguins. Available online: http://www.fphch.org/FR/education/Weiterbildung/faehigkeitsausweise/Impfen_und_Blutentnahme/Pages/default.aspx (accessed on 29 September 2018).
3. European Commission. Proposal for a Council Recommendation on Strengthened Cooperation against Vaccine Preventable Diseases. Available online: https://ec.europa.eu/health/sites/health/files/vaccination/docs/com2018_2442_en.pdf (accessed on 28 September 2018).
4. Le Conseil Fédéral Suisse. Ordonnance sur les Autorisations dans le Domaine des Médicaments (OAMéd). Available online: https://www.admin.ch/opc/fr/classified-compilation/20011780/index.html (accessed on 28 September 2018).
5. PharmaSuisse. La Vaccination Contre la Grippe—Un Service Proposé en Pharmacie sans Rendez-Vous. Available online: https://vaccinationenpharmacie.ch/assets/aktuelles/01-171031-grippeimfpung-pharmasuisse-fr.pdf (accessed on 28 September 2018).

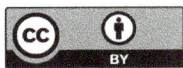

pharmacy

MDPI

Review

The Role of Community Pharmacists in Travel Health and Vaccination in Switzerland

Claudine Leuthold [1], Olivier Bugnon [2,3,4] and Jérôme Berger [2,3,4,*]

[1] PharmaSuisse, the Swiss Association of Pharmacists, CH-3097 Bern-Liebefeld, Switzerland; claudine.leuthold@pharmasuisse.org
[2] Community Pharmacy Centre, Department of Ambulatory Care and Community Medicine, University of Lausanne, CH-1011 Lausanne, Switzerland; olivier.bugnon@hospvd.ch
[3] Community Pharmacy Practice Research, School of pharmaceutical sciences, University of Geneva, CH-1206 Genève, Switzerland
[4] Community Pharmacy Practice Research, School of pharmaceutical sciences, University of Lausanne, CH-1206 Genève, Switzerland
* Correspondence: jerome.berger@hospvd.ch; Tel.: +41-21-314-48-43

Received: 7 November 2018; Accepted: 26 November 2018; Published: 29 November 2018

check for updates

Abstract: This review presents the Swiss strategy initiated over the last several years to implement vaccination by community pharmacists. National health authorities aimed to integrate community pharmacists in the National Vaccination Strategy (NVS) in order to increase the vaccination rate in the Swiss population. To support this aim, universities and the Swiss Association of Pharmacists developed pre- and post-graduate education programmes on vaccination for pharmacists. Finally, each Swiss canton (sovereign for health-related aspects) set proper regulations to authorize pharmacists to vaccinate and to determine which vaccines could be administered. As of September 2018, 19 cantons (out of 26) had authorized influenza vaccinations under the sole responsibility of an accredited community pharmacist. Additional vaccinations were available in 13 cantons (e.g., tick-borne encephalitis or hepatitis A, B, or A and B). Such implementation in other countries should follow a similar top-down (following a national strategy to improve vaccination coverage) and stepwise (starting with influenza to demonstrate the competencies of community pharmacists) strategy, supported by the development of research, education and accreditation. The development of health advice related to travels in community pharmacies should follow the same development in Switzerland. Currently, it offers the opportunity for strengthening travellers' safety, beyond vaccination issues.

Keywords: travel medicine; pharmacy; community; travel; practice; vaccination; Switzerland; education

1. Introduction

Until 2015, a prescription was required to authorize Swiss community pharmacists to supply vaccines, which were administered by other health professionals. This review presents the legal and practice changes that occurred in the last years to implement vaccination in community pharmacies and to include community pharmacists in the National Vaccination Strategy (NVS) from Swiss health authorities. This article also summarizes the activities, education, current situation, and legal frame of Swiss community pharmacists in the field of travel health and vaccination. It is based on reports from the heath authorities and from the national association of pharmacists (pharmaSuisse). Finally, it proposes future developments to strengthen the roles of community pharmacists in health services related to travel and vaccination.

2. Community Pharmacists and Travel Health

In Switzerland, any pharmacist has the basic skills to provide specific advice related to health promotion while traveling, in accordance with the responsibilities assigned by the Federal Law on Medical Professions [1]. This is an important activity, as 8.4 million Swiss citizens travel extensively (approximately 1.8 million trips outside Europe in 2017) [2]. This advice includes, for example, safe sex, sun protection, mosquito bite prevention, water purification or motion sickness treatment. To support this activity, pharmacists can provide sanitary materials, pharmacy kits or non-prescription medicines. In addition, pharmacists have to ensure the responsible use of antimalarial and anti-infective medicines, as well as vaccines, that they deliver under medical prescription. Their recommendations related to malaria and infectious disease risks are based on those issued by the Travel Medicine Centre of the University of Zurich and the Swiss Tropical and Public Health Institute of Basel. These are published by the Federal Office of Public Health (FOPH) [3], which is responsible for public health in Switzerland and develops Switzerland's health policies and contributes to ensuring that the country has an efficient and affordable healthcare system [4]. The practice recommendations issued by the FOPH are disseminated by two websites that can be used by community pharmacists, one for the public (www.safetravel.ch) and one for health professional (www.tropimed.ch). These websites display useful information related to travel health, as well as official recommendations adapted to the target audiences, completed with additional related information and maps.

3. Community Pharmacists and Vaccination

In addition to the activities related to health promotion while traveling that can be performed on a national level by any community pharmacist, some accredited pharmacists are authorized to administer some vaccines, e.g., to people seeking advice before travelling abroad (see Table 1). This accreditation depends on the canton where the community pharmacists are practising. Indeed, each Swiss canton is sovereign for health-related aspects: community pharmacists can be authorized or not to vaccinate and the list of vaccines they can administer varies among cantons. To be authorized to vaccinate in a canton where this practice is possible, a community pharmacist must undergo post-graduate education.

Table 1. Vaccinations authorized in community pharmacies, according to Swiss cantons (status in September 2018) [5].

Canton (Year of the Given Authorization to Perform Vaccination in Community Pharmacies)	Vaccinations Authorized in Community Pharmacies							
	Influenza	Tick-Borne Encephalitis	Hepatitis A	Hepatitis B	Hepatitis A and B	Measles, Mumps and Rubella	Human Papillomavirus	Diphtheria, Tetanus, and Pertussis
Lucerne (2017) Thurgau (2016)	+	+	+*	+*	+*	+*	+*	+*
Basel-Landschaft (2016)	+	+	+*	+*	+*	+*	-	-
Solothurn (2015)	+	+	+	+	+	+	-	-
Vaud (2016)	+	+	+*	+*	+*	+	-	-
Bern (2015), Graubünden (2016), Nidwalden (2017), Schaffhausen (2016), Schwyz (2016), Zug (2017), Zurich (2015)	+	+	+*	+*	+*	-	-	-
Fribourg (2015)	+	+	-	-	-	+	-	+
Basel-Stadt (2018)	+	+	+	+	+	-	-	-
Neuchâtel (2015)	+	+	-	-	-	+*	-	-
St. Gallen (2016)	+	+	-	-	-	-	-	-
Geneva (2016), Valais (2016), Jura (2016)	+	-	-	-	-	-	-	-

+: vaccination authorized in community pharmacy; +*: vaccination authorized in community pharmacy for the second dose, the first dose has to be administered by a physician; -: vaccination not authorized in community pharmacy.

The FOPH integrated pharmacists as potential actors and partners for vaccination in the NVS that was initiated from 2012 to 2017 [6]. This integration was based on the assessment of the influenza national vaccination campaigns performed in 2008 to 2012, which did not include community pharmacists [7]. This assessment showed that most of the goals of the campaign were not reached because of three main causes: (1). the vaccination rate of the various target groups decreased over the time; (2) the health professionals (mainly physicians) did not implement vaccinations in their daily practice; and (3) the "multiplier groups" did not include enough health professionals (the FOPH defined "multiplier groups" as physicians, cantonal health authorities, or media in charge of supporting and disseminating the health authorities' messages regarding vaccination). The community pharmacists were identified as able to reach the "healthy" population that had no regular contact with a general practitioner (GP). For example, in 2012, 34% of Swiss citizens above 15 years old declared to have had no appointment with a GP in the previous 12 months [8]. In addition, community pharmacists were considered as a potential "multiplier group" to increase the vaccination coverage in the Swiss population. Indeed, there is approximately one community pharmacy for every 4700 people in Switzerland [9]. Another element that advocated towards the inclusion of community pharmacists in the NVS was that the FOPH wanted to promote the use of the electronic vaccination plan (www.myvaccines.ch); thirty percent of community pharmacies were already subscribers of this website [10].

Based on the aim of the FOPH to integrate community pharmacists in the NVS and on foreign experiences of vaccination services in community pharmacies, the Swiss Association of Pharmacists (pharmaSuisse) initiated a post-graduate educational programme to train and accredit community pharmacists for vaccination. Based on American and Portuguese experiences, a Swiss post-graduate training certificate named (in French) "Certificat de formation complémentaire FPH Vaccination et prélèvements sanguins (Foederatio Pharmaceutica Helvetiae)" [11] was created in 2011. The first community pharmacists were accredited in 2012.

Following the recommendations of the FOPH to encourage vaccination in community pharmacies and the post-graduate training in vaccination for community pharmacists, some cantons began to authorize vaccination by trained and accredited community pharmacists in 2015. This required changes in the Swiss laws to allow community pharmacists to administer a vaccine without a prior medical prescription. Then, each canton had to establish proper regulations to determine which vaccines could be administered and which facilities were required on the premises of community pharmacies to perform vaccination.

As of September 2018, the situation in the 26 Swiss cantons was as follows: six cantons (Aargau, Appenzell Inner-Rhodes, Appenzell Outer Rhodes, Glarus, Obwalden, and Uri) had not yet authorized vaccination in community pharmacies, one canton (Ticino) had authorized vaccination only when prescribed by a physician, and 19 cantons had authorized vaccinations under the sole responsibility of an accredited community pharmacist (see Table 1). In the cantons that authorized vaccinations by accredited community pharmacists, influenza vaccination was the first to be available, and it was followed by other vaccinations in 16 cantons. Age limits have to be considered for vaccination in community pharmacies; this is only approved for people older than 16 years old (18 years old in Basel-Stadt and Basel-Landschaft), and two cantons (Geneva and Valais) do not permit vaccination of people over 65 years old. Currently, more than 1400 community pharmacists (out of 5300) are accredited and approximately 700 pharmacies (out of 1800) are available for vaccination [5].

4. Education of Community Pharmacists related to Travel Health and Vaccination

Three different universities (Basel, Geneva, and Zürich) offer a full curriculum for pharmacy students in Switzerland. Pre-graduate training objectives are defined at the national level by FOPH in concordance with the Federal Law on Medical Professions [12]. The national vaccination schemes as well as the responsible use of the vaccines registered on the Swiss market are included in the objectives. This is the common minimum base related to vaccination that has to be taught in each university. Beside this, each university completes its lessons and learning objectives according to the needs of local community pharmacists. For example, at the University of Geneva, 4 h on health advices related to travel in community pharmacy (e.g., malaria prevention or travelling with medicines) and 4 h on vaccination (e.g., vaccination schemes, vaccination booklet, and advice on vaccination in community pharmacy) are taught to master students in pharmacy. In addition, pre-graduate courses are currently reviewed according to revised national learning objectives for community pharmacists. Hence, injection and blood sample collection techniques are or will be included in pre-graduate courses. For example, such courses are already included in the curriculum of the University of Basel and will be included at the University of Geneva in the near future.

4.1. Post-Graduate Education in Travel Health

There is no mandatory post-graduate education related to travel health for community pharmacists in Switzerland. However, there are various continuous trainings that are available for pharmacists: e.g., the "Swiss Tropical and Public Health Institute—International Short Course on Travellers' Health", which gives relevant and updated information to assess travel-related health problems and to give preventive pre-travel advice, with a focus on tropical diseases, vaccination and prophylaxis; or the (in French) "Journée Romande de Médecine des Voyages", which gives an annual update on various topics related to travel medicine. In addition, Swiss community pharmacists can participate in international trainings, such as the Conference of the International Society of Travel Medicine (CISTM), which is organized every two years [13].

4.2. Post-Graduate Education in Vaccination

Currently, each canton that authorizes community pharmacists to vaccinate requires pharmacists to hold an accreditation named (in French) "Certificat de formation complémentaire FPH (Foederatio Pharmaceutica Helvetiae) Vaccination et prélèvements sanguins", that demonstrates their skills in vaccination, injection and blood samples techniques. This training lasts four and a half days. It includes theoretical and practical lessons, both with face-to-face and e-learning courses, followed by a complete "Adult basic life support and automated external defibrillation" (BLS AED). To renew his accreditation and maintain the authorization to vaccinate, each community pharmacist has to complete a minimum of one day of training related to vaccination at least every two years. Swiss or international continuous education related to travel medicine can be recognized as a part of this mandatory training [11].

5. Studies Related to Travel Health and Vaccination in Swiss Community Pharmacies

To our knowledge, no national study concerning activities in community pharmacies related to travels has been conducted in Switzerland.

Regarding vaccination, a national observational study, based on the voluntary reporting of influenza vaccination by community pharmacists registered on a paying web platform (www. vaccinationenpharmacie.ch), has been realized in the last influenza season (from 1 December 2017 to 31 January 2018) [14]. The results showed that 12,490 vaccinations were administered with written informed consent by accredited pharmacists active in 472 authorized pharmacies. A statistical extrapolation performed based on this study estimated that almost 20,000 influenza vaccinations were administered in authorized pharmacies over the same period [15]. The main limitation of this study is related to the fact that its results are based on the voluntary reporting of vaccinations on a paying web platform that is not systematically used. Hence, the total number of influenza vaccinations performed in Swiss community pharmacies over the same period is probably much larger.

Other studies related to vaccination in community pharmacies are currently underway at local levels (e.g., in the French-speaking canton of Vaud).

6. Discussion

Improving vaccination coverage by developing and implementing national vaccination plans is a major public health issue [16]. A global strategy has been conducted by health authorities to increase access to vaccination in the last several years in Switzerland [6]. Vaccination in Swiss community pharmacies has been identified as a mean to sustain this strategy, as it represents an option for adults who want to protect themselves, as well as their communities, and who do not have a referent GP or who do not want to visit their GP. This convenient access to vaccination is not only recognized in Switzerland and has already been implemented in several countries (e.g., Australia, Canada, Portugal, or the United States) [17]. Such strategies have to be adapted to each national context to be successful. In Switzerland, it considered the specificities regarding the different roles of health authorities at the national and cantonal levels. The national strategy recommended facilitating the contribution of community pharmacies to implement vaccination and defined the conditions and objectives for such involvement. Then, each canton determined the practical aspects to adapt the implementation to their particular context. Compared to a fully national strategy, this probably allowed to implement earlier vaccination in community pharmacies and to broaden the vaccines that can be administered by pharmacists in some cantons. This type of implementation process combining top-down and stepwise approaches (starting with influenza vaccination to demonstrate the competencies and impact of community pharmacists) can inspire other countries, especially federal ones. In addition, the parallel and complementarity development of pre- and post-graduate training programmes conducted by universities and professional associations of pharmacists seems to be an important element in such a strategy. Further developments in the continuous education of community pharmacists remain to be implemented. Indeed, community pharmacists are gaining more and more experience in vaccination. Hence, their needs related to the mandatory training required to renew their accreditation will certainly evolve. Advice related to travel health in community pharmacies has not yet been included in similar national and cantonal strategies. The increasing number of travels abroad by Swiss citizens [2] might lead to the development of new activities in community pharmacies, related to this specific public health issue, as in the United Kingdom [18]. Currently, this activity represents a good opportunity for strengthening travellers' safety, beyond vaccination issues.

7. Conclusions

Top-down and stepwise strategies supported by education, accreditation and practice research activities showed to be effective to implement vaccination by Swiss community pharmacists. To finalize this implementation, continuous education should be adapted to meet new needs from community pharmacists experienced in vaccination. In addition, research should be supported to assess the effectiveness of community pharmacists, e.g., on vaccination coverage. Similar strategies should be conducted in other countries to involve community pharmacists in vaccination. In Switzerland, this could serve as a model to strengthen the role of community pharmacists in other public health developments.

Author Contributions: For research articles with several authors, a short paragraph specifying their individual contributions must be provided. The following statements should be used "Conceptualization, C.L., O.B. and J.B.; Methodology, J.B.; Formal Analysis, C.L. and J.B.; Investigation, C.L.; Resources, C.L., O.B. and J.B.; Data Curation, C.L.; Writing-Original Draft Preparation, C.L. and J.B.; Writing-Review & Editing, J.B.; Supervision, O.B and J.B; please turn to the CRediT taxonomy for the term explanation. Authorship must be limited to those who have contributed substantially to the work reported.

Funding: This research received no external funding.

Conflicts of Interest: The authors declare no conflict of interest.

References

1. Le Conseil Fédéral Suisse. Loi Fédérale sur les Professions Médicales Universitaires (LPMéd) (only in German, French and Italian). Available online: https://www.admin.ch/opc/fr/classified-compilation/20040265/index.html (accessed on 15 October 2018).
2. Federal Statistical Office FSO. Trips with Overnight Stays. Available online: https://www.bfs.admin.ch/bfs/en/home/statistics/tourism/travel-behaviour/overnight-stays.html (accessed on 23 November 2018).
3. Office Fédéral de la Santé Publique OFSP. Santé-Voyages: Vaccinations et Mesures Antipaludiques (only in German, French and Italian). Available online: https://www.bag.admin.ch/bag/fr/home/gesund-leben/gesundheitsfoerderung-und-praevention/impfungen-prophylaxe/reiseimpfungen.html (accessed on 18 October 2018).
4. Federal Office of Public Health FOPH. Taking Health to Heart. Tasks and Goals. Available online: https://www.bag.admin.ch/bag/en/home/das-bag/auftrag-ziele.html (accessed on 18 October 2018).
5. PharmaSuisse. Vaccination en Pharmacie (only in German and French for Registered Pharmacists). Available online: www.vaccinationenpharmacie.ch (accessed on 18 October 2018).
6. Federal Office of Public Health FOPH. National Vaccination Strategy (NVS). Available online: https://www.bag.admin.ch/bag/en/home/strategie-und-politik/nationale-gesundheitsstrategien/nationale-strategie-impfungen-nsi.html (accessed on 18 October 2018).
7. Office Fédéral de la Santé Publique OFSP. Rapports D'évaluation sur les Maladies Transmissibles: Evaluation de la Stratégie de Communication Pour la Prévention de la Grippe Saisonnière 2008-2012 (only in German and French). Available online: https://www.bag.admin.ch/bag/fr/home/das-bag/publikationen/evaluationsberichte/evalber-uebertragbare-krankheiten.html (accessed on 18 October 2018).
8. Observatoire Suisse de la Santé OBSAN; Office Fédéral de la Statistique. Consultations Chez le Médecin Généraliste ou de Famille (only in German and French). Available online: https://www.obsan.admin.ch/fr/indicateurs/consultations-chez-le-medecin-generaliste-ou-de-famille (accessed on 18 October 2018).
9. Office Fédéral de la Statistique. Système de Santé: Autres Prestataires (only in German and French). Available online: https://www.bfs.admin.ch/bfs/fr/home/statistiques/sante/systeme-sante/autres-prestataires.html (accessed on 18 October 2018).
10. Leuthold, C. Personal Communication. PharmaSuisse: Bern, Switzerland, 5 June 2018.
11. Foederatio Pharmaceutica Helvetiae. Formation Postgrade FPH—Vaccination et Prélèvements Sanguins (only in German and French). Available online: http://www.fphch.org/FR/education/Weiterbildung/faehigkeitsausweise/Impfen_und_Blutentnahme/Pages/default.aspx (accessed on 18 October 2018).
12. Office Fédéral de la Santé Publique OFSP. Catalogue des Objectifs de Formation en Pharmacie (only in German and French). Available online: https://www.bag.admin.ch/dam/bag/fr/dokumente/berufe-gesundheitswesen/medizinalberufe/eidg-pruefungen-universitaerer-medizinalberufe/pharmazie/lernzielkatalog-pharmazie1.pdf.download.pdf/lernzielkatalog-pharmazie-version-2.pdf (accessed on 18 October 2018).
13. International Society of Travel Medicine ISTM. Available online: http://www.istm.org/ (accessed on 18 October 2018).
14. PharmaSuisse. Collecte de Données par les Pharmacies Concernant la Campagne de Vaccination Antigrippale 2017/2018 (only in German and French). Available online: https://vaccinationenpharmacie.ch/assets/kampagnenmaterial/publikationen-und-datenerhebung-f/6-datenerhebung-grippeimpfaktion-2017-18-fr-v2.pdf (accessed on 18 October 2018).
15. PharmaSuisse. Impfen in der Apotheke: Bestandsaufnahme und Erfahrungen der Apotheken (only in German and French). Available online: https://vaccinationenpharmacie.ch/assets/aktuelles/7-pharmasuisse-studie-impfen-2018-08-16.pdf (accessed on 18 October 2018).
16. European Commission. Live, Work, Travel in the EU/Public Health/Vaccination. Available online: https://ec.europa.eu/health/vaccination/overview_en (accessed on 23 November 2018).

17. Vaccines Europe. Improving Access and Convenience to Vaccination. Available online: https://www.vaccineseurope.eu/wp-content/uploads/2018/06/VE-Flu-Vaccination-Access-Pharmacies-0506018-FIN-FIN.pdf (accessed on 23 November 2018).
18. Evans, D. Impact of Pharmacy Based Travel Medicine with the Evolution of Pharmacy Practice in the UK. *Pharmacy* **2018**, *6*, 64. [CrossRef] [PubMed]

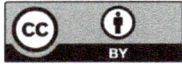

Review

The Role of Pharmacists in Travel Medicine in South Africa

Lee Baker

Amayeza Info Services, Johannesburg 1709, South Africa; lee@amayeza-info.co.za

Received: 16 June 2018; Accepted: 17 July 2018; Published: 19 July 2018

Abstract: Worldwide, pharmacists, who are the most accessible health-care providers, are playing an ever increasing role in travel medicine, assisting travelers in taking the necessary precautions to ensure safe and healthy travel. This article looks at the situation in South Africa, and how pharmacists are performing these functions within the legal constraints of the Medicines and Related Substances Act 101 of 1965, which prevents pharmacists from prescribing many of the travel vaccines and medications. The scope of practice in community pharmacies increased since the successful down-scheduling of some of the antimalarials, allowing pharmacists to supply the many travelers who frequently travel to neighboring countries. As in many other countries, travel medicine in South Africa is currently thwart with products that are out of stock, and a number of temporary guidelines were put in place to deal with these. Ways to facilitate expanding the role of pharmacists in travel medicine in South Africa need to be further explored.

Keywords: pharmacists; travel medicine; malaria; malaria prophylaxis; South Africa; schedules

1. Pharmacist Prescribing in South Africa

There are 3370 community pharmacists in South Africa [1], and they potentially have a very important role to play in travel medicine in South Africa, especially with regards to malaria, as there are many malaria-stricken areas within a couple of hours' travel from people's homes, which are often visited on weekends. There is also a significant migrant population from neighboring countries that come to South Africa seeking work, and who go home in December (the height of malaria season). Pharmacists are the most accessible health-care professionals, and are, therefore, frequently consulted regarding malaria prophylaxis and other travel health matters. In spite of this, the formal role of pharmacists in travel medicine is in its infancy when compared to some countries such as Canada [2]. This is mainly due to legislature which prevents pharmacists from prescribing or dispensing (without a prescription) any medicine above schedule 2. Medicines in South Africa are scheduled from 0–8, which determines the rules relating to the sale thereof, with schedule 0 (S0) sold in supermarkets, and S3 and up on prescription only. Most travel vaccines are schedule 4 [3].

In addition to the scope of practice of a pharmacist, a pharmacist with the Primary Care Drug Therapy (PCDT) qualification and a Section 22A (15) permit issued by the Director General of Health is permitted to diagnose, treat, and supply medicines following the Primary Health Care Standard Treatment Guidelines and the list of approved medicines, as an authorized prescriber [4].

Section 22A(15) of the Medicines and Related Substances Act (Act 101 of 1965) states that the Director General issues Section 22A(15) permits after consultation with the South African Pharmacy Council (SAPC). Primary Care Drug Therapy (PCDT) permits are issued with a list of conditions and medications that the pharmacist in possession of the permit may prescribe and dispense. This list is in line with the Department of Health's latest Essential Medicines List. This section reads as follows: "Notwithstanding anything to the contrary contained in this section, the Director General may, after consultation with the Interim Pharmacy Council of South Africa as referred to in Section 2 of the

Pharmacy Act, 1974 (Act 53 of 1974), issue a permit to any person or organization performing a health service, authorizing such person or organization to acquire, possess, use, or supply any specified schedule 1, schedule 2, schedule 3, schedule 4, or schedule 5 substance, and such permit shall be subject to such conditions as the Director General may determine [3]." Any application for the scheduling of medicines for this purpose, or for access in terms of Section 22A(15) of the Act should, therefore, use the most recent set of Standard Treatment Guidelines/Essential Medicines List (STG/EML) for Primary Health Care (PHC) issued by the National Department of Health as a starting point, wherever appropriate. The PHC STG/EML is intended to guide the practice of medical practitioners and nurses at PHC facilities in the public sector. Pediatric vaccines against polio, tuberculosis, diphtheria, tetanus, pertussis, hepatitis B, *haemophilus influenzae* type b, measles, pneumococcal, and rotavirus infections are on the Primary Health Care Essential Medicines List, and pharmacists with this Section 22A(15) permit can administer them. The human papillomavirus (HPV) vaccine and the influenza vaccines are also on this list [5]. However, none of the travel vaccines are on this list, and the pharmacist cannot, therefore, prescribe and administer them.

2. Pharmacist Activity in Travel Medicine

Currently, 10 pharmacists are members of the South African Society of Travel Medicine (SASTM), and they have all completed the Travel Medicine Course offered once a year by the SASTM, and accredited by the Witwatersrand University. Pharmacists and nurses may only apply to do this course if they have a medical practitioner overseeing them who has either done the course or will do the course with them [6]. This is a very comprehensive course, which equips them with the knowledge they need to be able to offer travel health of the highest standard. This entitles them to apply for a yellow fever license, which allows them to administer these vaccines if they are prescribed by a doctor. Although they cannot prescribe and dispense the necessary vaccines and medicines, they usually work closely with doctors or travel clinics, and play an important role in counseling [3,6]. Most community pharmacists actively counsel travelers on a daily basis, particularly with respect to malaria prophylaxis. Topics that they give advice on, and where possible, products to minimize risks include, traveler's diarrhea, jetlag, motion sickness, altitude sickness, and prophylaxis of venous thromboembolism [7].

Very few pharmacists currently run their own travel clinics because of the constraints; however, many of the bigger pharmacy groups have started clinics that administer childhood vaccines, and they would be in a good position to open up travel clinics. A few community pharmacists completed the SASTM course and worked under the supervision of a doctor. They are in small rural towns, and they play a very important role.

Two pharmacists, who did the course, worked in a medicine information center, the only privately run one in South Africa. Only one is still employed by the center. Various services are offered, with two of them being a malaria information line and a vaccine information line. Both these services are utilized by health-care professionals, as well as by members of the public. The medicine information center is the Amayeza Info Centre www.amayeza-info.co.za.

Pharmacists have access to a number of resources to assist them with travel health. Those that are members of the SASTM have access to Travax www.travax.nhs.uk and anyone can access the Centers for Disease Control and Prevention (CDC) website for travel health https://wwwnc.cdc.gov/travel, and the World Health Organization (WHO) website for travel and health www.who.int/topics/travel/en/. South African information is available from the National Institute of Communicable Diseases www.nicd.ac.za and the South African National Travel Health Network www.santhnet.co.za.

The current president of the SASTM is a pharmacist, and, in her private capacity, she also sits on the South African Malaria Elimination Committee (SAMEC), which is a committee, made up of experts in the field of malaria, that advises the National Department of Health on malaria. This committee is involved in drawing up the Guidelines for the Treatment of Malaria in South Africa 2018 [8] and the South African Guidelines for the Prevention of Malaria 2017 [9], as well as being instrumental in getting intravenous (IV) artesunate registered in South Africa, and some of the chemoprophylaxis products down-scheduled.

3. Antimalarials through Pharmacies

For a medicine to be rescheduled in South Africa, the manufacturer is required to make a submission to the scheduling committee of the Medicines Control Council (MCC), which is now the South African Health Products Regulatory Authority (SAHPRA). In order to make antimalarials more accessible to the public, in the hopes that this would reduce the number of imported malaria cases in South Africa as the country moves toward malaria elimination, the SAMEC approached both the manufacturers and the scheduling committee with a motivation to down-schedule some of the antimalarials. After a number of years of trying to get them down-scheduled to enable a pharmacist to dispense them without a prescription, this was recently achieved. Two years ago, in March 2016, doxycycline [10], and in November 2017, atovaquone-proguanil [11] were cleared to be given out by pharmacists without a prescription. This has enormous benefit for the many travelers who only became aware of the need to obtain antimalarials close to the time of the planned trip, and who did not have sufficient time to arrange for a prescription. In order to ensure that pharmacists are adequately knowledgeable to recommend and dispense these antimalarials, a number of continuing professional development (CPD) talks were given, as well as articles being published in pharmacy and medical journals [12,13].

In the last two years, both South Africa and its neighboring countries have experienced a surge in malaria cases [14]. Namibia experienced four times more cases in 2017 compared to 2015, and incidence rates in Zambia, Mozambique, and Malawi were between 286 and 381 per 1000 people in 2016. Mozambique, which is a popular destination for South Africans, and is also one of the countries from where many of South Africa's migrant workers come, has between six and eight million cases a year. South Africa's cases increased from about 5000 cases in 2016 to more than 30,000 cases in 2017 [15]. It is hoped that improving accessibility to antimalarials will result in more travelers taking them, and in a reduction in the number of cases.

4. Future Developments

In terms of the Regulations relating to the registration of the Specialities of Pharmacists, Council recognizes Master's Programs for registration as specialists. There are two specialities currently registrable with Council, i.e., Radio-pharmacy and Clinical Pharmacokinetics [16]. The way forward would be to have travel medicine registered as a speciality. It will then be possible to design a course that will allow pharmacists to prescribe vaccines and medicines appropriate for travel (as the PCDT course only allows them to prescribe for primary care).

5. Current Challenges

Travel medicine in general, not specific to pharmacists, saw many challenges in the last year. Many of the travel vaccines and antimalarials were out of stock for months at a time; there is only one manufacturer of pediatric atovaquone-proguanil, and they were out of stock, as was the case with mefloquine, whereas doxycycline cannot be given to children under the age of eight, resulting in no antimalarials available for young children. Vaccine shortages are a worldwide problem; many parts of the world have a yellow-fever vaccine shortage, which South Africa fortunately does not. Both hepatitis A and B vaccines are in short supply, which led to the development of guidelines to deal with these [17,18].

Despite these challenges, travel medicine is alive and well in South Africa, and it is hoped that pharmacists will play an even bigger role in the near future. In a study published earlier this year, clinical outcomes and traveler satisfaction with a pharmacy-based travel clinic was evaluated in Alberta, Canada. Traveler satisfaction was reported as very high with infrequent health issues during travel, and the majority of those who did experience health problems felt that they were adequately prepared

Pharmacy **2018**, *6*, 68

to cope with them [2]. These results support an earlier study done in Scotland [19]. Such evidence is important to promote continued expansion of pharmacists' scope in this area, and it is hoped that similar results will be seen in South Africa in the not-too-distant future.

Funding: This research received no external funding.

Acknowledgments: I would like to acknowledge Prof Larry Goodyer for assisting me with the format of this article.

Conflicts of Interest: The author declares no conflict of interest.

References

1. Statistics of Registered Persons and Organisations. 2018. Available online: https://www.pharmcouncil.co.za/B_Statistics.asp (accessed on 22 May 2018).
2. Houle, S.K.D.; Bascom, C.S.; Rosenthal, M.M. Clinical outcomes and satisfaction with a pharmacist-managed travel clinic in Alberta, Canada. *Travel Med. Infect. Dis.* **2018**, *23*, 21–26. [CrossRef] [PubMed]
3. SAHPRA. Acts, Regulations and Government Notices. 101 Medicines and Related Substances Act 101. 1965. Available online: http://www.mccza.com/Publications (accessed on 22 May 2018).
4. SAHPRA. Scheduling of Substances for Prescribing by Authorised Prescribers. Available online: http://www.mccza.com/documents/fb489cf12.37_Scheduling_for_Prescribing_by_Authorised_Prescribers_Mar14_v1.pdf (accessed on 18 July 2018).
5. Standard Treatment Guidelines and Essential Medicines List for South Africa Primary Health Care Level 2014. Available online: http://www.health.gov.za/index.php/component/phocadownload/category/285-phc (accessed on 22 May 2018).
6. Travel Medicine Course. The South African Society of Travel Medicine. Available online: www.sastm.org.za (accessed on 15 June 2018).
7. Meyer, J.C.; Nkonde, K.; Schellack, N. Travel medicine: An overview. *S. Afr. Pharm. J.* **2017**, *84*, 19–28.
8. Guidelines for the Treatment of Malaria in South Africa. 2018. Available online: www.Santhnet.co.za (accessed on 14 June 2018).
9. South African Guidelines for the Prevention of Malaria. Available online: https://www.google.com/url?sa=t&rct=j&q=&esrc=s&source=web&cd=1&ved=0ahUKEwiLr83_lKrcAhVU_GEKHUp0AicQFggwMAA&url=http%3A%2F%2Fwww.nicd.ac.za%2Fwp-content%2Fuploads%2F2017%2F09%2FGuidelines-South-African-Guidelines-for-the-Prevention-of-Malaria-2017-final.pdf&usg=AOvVaw2JINqVj7gggDq4uz3FVVQv (accessed on 14 June 2018).
10. Government Gazette. 15 March 2016. Volume 609, No. 39815. Available online: www.gpwonline.co.za (accessed on 13 February 2018).
11. Gouws, J.C. Registrar of Medicines. Communication to Industry. Medicine Control Council. Department of Health. Available online: www.mccza.com/Publications/DownloadDoc/5587 (accessed on 13 July 2018).
12. Baker, L. Malaria prophylaxis—Can we conquer the 'mighty' parasite? *S. Afr. Pharm. J.* **2018**, *85*, 48–54.
13. Parker, S. Malaria drug: Rescheduling treatment adherence. *Med. Chron.* **2018**, *3*, 2–3.
14. Blumberg, L.; Frean, J. Malaria reduces globally but rebounds across southern Africa. *S. Afr. J. Infect. Dis.* **2017**, *32*, 3–4.
15. SADC Malaria Report 2017. Available online: https://www.google.com/url?sa=t&rct=j&q=&esrc=s&source=web&cd=1&ved=0ahUKEwiv_rXphqrcAhXVdt4KHeg9AsEQFggrMAA&url=http%3A%2F%2Fwww.health.gov.za%2Findex.php%2Fcomponent%2Fphocadownload%2Fcategory%2F422-malaria-2017%3Fdownload%3D2529%3Asadc-malaria-report-2017&usg=AOvVaw0Dwli79m7Ik4jj88aZkT7R (accessed on 18 July 2018).
16. Specialities in Pharmacy. Available online: https://www.pharmcouncil.co.za/B_Edu_AccOfCourses.asp (accessed on 22 May 2018).
17. Hepatitis A Vaccination in Adults—Temporary Recommendations. Published July 2017 PHE Publications Gateway Number: 2017175. Available online: https://www.gov.uk/government/publications/hepatitis-a-infection-prevention-and-control-guidance (accessed on 15 June 2018).

18. Hepatitis B Vaccination in Adults and Children: Temporary Recommendations from 21 August 2017. Published 21 August 2017 PHE Publications Gateway Number: 2017256. Available online: https://assets.publishing.service.gov.uk/government/uploads/system/uploads/attachment_data/file/639145/Hepatitis_B_vaccine_recommendations_during_supply_constraints.pdf (accessed on 15 June 2018).
19. Hind, C.; Bond, C.; Lee, A.J.; van Teijlingen, E. Travel medicine services from community pharmacy: Evaluation of a pilot service. *Pharm. J.* **2018**, *281*, 625–632.

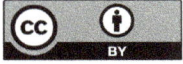

pharmacy

MDPI

Review

Impact of Pharmacy Based Travel Medicine with the Evolution of Pharmacy Practice in the UK

Derek Evans

FRPharmS, FRGS, MFTM RCPS, Independent Prescriber, 58 The Nurseries, Langstone, Wales NP18 2NT, UK;
d.p.evans@btinternet.com

Received: 10 May 2018; Accepted: 5 July 2018; Published: 9 July 2018

check for
updates

Abstract: Background: Pharmacy has utilised the changes in legislation since 2000 to increase the range and supply function of services such as travel health to travellers. With the number of travellers leaving the UK and trying new destinations there is an increasing need for more travel health provision. Working models: The models of supply of a travel health service vary according to the size of the corporate body. The large multiples can offer assessment via a specialist nurse or doctor service and then supply through the pharmacy. Others will undertake an onsite risk assessment and supply through the pharmacist. The sole Internet suppliers of medication have been reviewed and the assessment standards questioned following survey and inspection. Education: There is no dedicated pharmacist-training programme in advanced level travel health. As a consequence one academic institution allows pharmacists to train on a multidisciplinary course to obtain an academic membership. With training for travel health not being mandatory for any travel health supply function the concern is raised with standards of care. Future: There is a consultation paper on the removal of travel vaccines from NHS supply due to be decided in the future. If these vaccines are removed then they will provide a greater demand on pharmacy services. Discussion: The starting of a travel health service can be made without any additional training and remains unregulated, giving cause for concern to the supply made to the traveller. Conclusions: Pharmacies in the UK offer a range of options for supplying travel health services; however these need to be with improved mandatory training and supply.

Keywords: travel medicine; health; pharmacist; pharmacy; vaccinations; prescribing and education

1. Introduction

This is a review of the development of the practice of pharmacy in the UK developing from the legal changes that occurred in the 2000s to include modern working models and specialist eduction that is available to pharmacists.

In the UK, prior to 2000 the role of the pharmacist was that of the traditional supply function against the supply of a prescription and the sale of over the counter products (OTC). Within the UK the legislation is defined in 3 legal categories of medicines, prescription only (POM)—only supplied against a doctors or dentists prescription (private and National Health Service (NHS)); pharmacy only medicines (PM)—only supplied from a licensed pharmacy in the presence of a pharmacist and OTC products. At this time there was no legislation that allowed pharmacists to provide routine or travel vaccinations or to supply POMs without a relevant prescription.

With changes to both the legal supply of POMs and the increasing requirement to use pharmacist's clinical skills then evolvement of influenza vaccination was introduced. This led onto the consideration of travel health health services from a pharmacy, by a pharmacist, to become established.

The changes to a nationally funded travel health service remain under scrutiny and with increasing numbers of patients travelling abroad annually (+5%) and +27% intending to to travel a country they have never visited before [1] the NHS is reviewing the current funding of these services.

2. Legislative Changes

In 1998 the NHS reviewed the medicines that where be allowed to be supplied on a prescription. This review included the removal of chloroquine for malaria prophylaxis and the change to PM status allowing it to be purchased from pharmacies, (Figure 1). The NHS continues to supply free of charge to all travellers' vaccines against hepatitis A, typhoid, diphtheria/tetanus/polio and cholera from surgery that is contracted to provide vaccinations. All other vaccinations remained on a private supply along with the antimalarials.

In 2000 following lobbying from the Royal College of Nurses (RCN) for group protocols to supply national immunisation services, the law was changed to allow the supply of medication by healthcare professionals using Patient Group Directions [2].

At the same time-work was underway to allow a new category of prescribers to be formed. This became known as supplementary prescribing, which was originally given to practice and district nurses working alongside a doctor to reduce the workload [3]. A supplementary prescriber was a healthcare professional who had the authority to supply a range of previously agreed drugs according to an agreed clinical management plan.

With the increase in clinical knowledge and skills being taught and applied to other healthcare professions the role of independent prescriber was created in 2006, which included pharmacists [4]. This role allowed a pharmacist, with a formal qualification in independent prescribing to be able to write diagnose, treat and write prescriptions. The ethical area of competence is unregulated and such prescribers a can legally write a prescription that may include schedule 2 Controlled Drugs [5].

A major change in the law occurred in 2012 with the introduction of the Human Medicines Regulations [6]. This allowed the widening of the range of medication that could be supplied under a PGD allowing more services to be created. Additional NHS regulations introduced at the same time allowed the concept of a new style of pharmacy, that of the at distance or "postal service" pharmacies, where a pharmacy could make an online sale or supply of a prescription without face to face contact with the patient. Alongside these regulations came the new standards of pharmacy premises which included the minimum design standards for every pharmacy to have a their own consultation room to provide services.

With the UK Government reviewing the impact of annual influenza absences and the pressure for new roles to be allowed to pharmacy the first pharmacy flu vaccination services were introduced in 2007 as a private service utilising PGDs. This continued until 2015 when it was extended and included as a pharmacy NHS funded service.

Alongside the provision of seasonal influenza vaccinations other vaccination services supplied by PGDs and Pharmacist Independent Prescriber (PIPs) evolved such as travel vaccinations and the supply of antimalarials for prophylaxis. With the austerity measures imposed on public spending private clinical services were considered as a part solution to maintaining financial solvency.

In late 2017 the PHE was tasked with a consultation between professionals to consider if the total withdrawal of all vaccines for pre-travel should be removed from the NHS [7] and made private supply only.

The significance of the changes to practice working at a faster rate than legislative changes has led to the introduction of support networks for pharmacists providing travel health service using telemedicine or at distance triage services completed by a nurse or doctor [8].

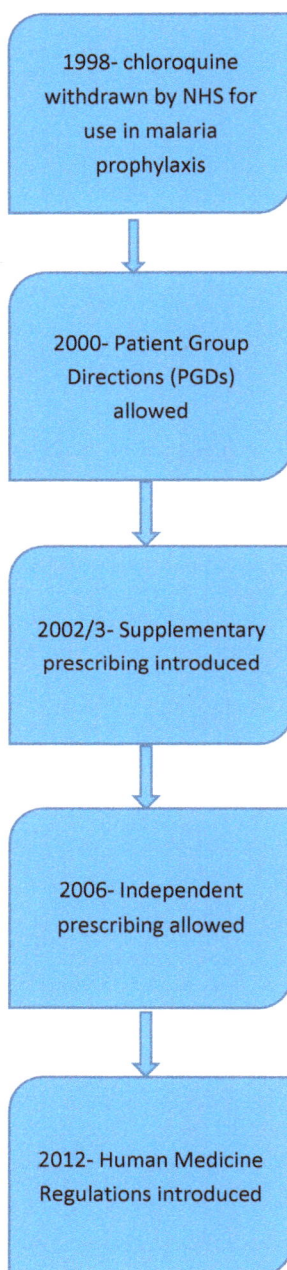

Figure 1. Key legislative changes allowing pharmacists to practice travel medicine.

3. Models of Working Practices

Within the pharmacy population in the UK, 49.2% of pharmacies are owned by groups and termed large multiples. Examples of these include Boots, Lloyds, Well, Rowlands and the supermarket groups of Asda, Morrisons and Tesco. Other smaller independents provide 12.4% and the remainder is made up small chains (<3 outlets) and independents 38.4% of the market [9].

Access to travel health or medicine services is varied and one type of model includes a risk assessment being completed externally by a doctor, nurse or pharmacist and then the vaccination or anti-malarial supply being authorised by either a private prescription or directed to a pharmacist through a Patient Specific Direction (PSD). (A PSD is a formal arrangement, which allows a doctor or independent prescriber to direct the supply of vaccination through another healthcare professional to a patient).

Other pharmacies, allow an online booking service to be made with one of its selected stores (not all stores are included) for a risk assessment lasting up to 40 min. The clinical support and backup is provided by a nurse led service to which the pharmacist can refer. The pharmacist can administer the vaccinations and supply the medication at the appointment.

The UK legislation differs at this point regarding the regulation of the standards of practice between solely organised pharmacist clinics and those by other healthcare professions. The regulating body in England, the Care Quality Commission (CQC) [10] regulates the standards to be applied in nurse or doctor led clinics; whilst the General Pharmaceutical Council (GPhC) regulates the standards in pharmacies. In 2017 the joint regulators investigated online prescribing to patients. The report highlighted significant areas of failure between some online prescribers and those in a patient-facing scenario [11]. A previous study evaluating the supply of atovaquone/proguanil through online prescribing highlighted that potential questions were no addressed such as previous ADR to the drugs (59%) or the length of stay in the malarial area (50%) [12].

A small independent survey study in 2018 concluded that a pharmacy travel health service was well accepted by patients and met their needs, providing a value for money service [13].

4. Travel Health Education

With the supply of POM medication made by pharmacists either under a PGD or as an Independent Prescriber the professional expectation is that the standard of training to use these preparations should be of the a similar standard at an advanced level. Within the UK there is no legal requirement to have received any formal advanced level training before using a PGD and whilst an Independent Prescriber qualifies in a defined area of competence, they are legally allowed to prescribe any medicinal product outside of their competence, including controlled drugs.

To ensure that basic immunisation is practiced correctly the GPhC in alliance with the Royal College of Nursing and Public Health England have published a document that lists the national minimum standards and core curriculum for immunisation training for registered healthcare practitioners [14].

For those pharmacists who do elect to undertake extended training there are ranges of courses in travel health that are shared with other professions allowing an equality between practitioners. Examples of this can be found at the centres of excellence of in London, Liverpool and Glasgow. Details of the courses available to pharmacists are seen in Table 1, an overview suggests that pharmacy professional courses are of a basic level and many of the advanced level courses are restricted to registered doctors and nurses only.

Table 1. Travel health training and education available to pharmacists in UK.

Institution	Travel Medicine Post-Graduate Course Available to Pharmacist	Formal Professional Accreditation
Faculty of Travel Medicine (FTM) of the Royal College of Physicians and Surgeons (Glasgow)	Diploma in Travel Medicine (12–15 months)	Membership of Faculty of Travel Medicine of RCPS
	Foundation in Travel Medicine (6 months) https://rcpsg.ac.uk/travel-medicine/education	None
London School of Hygiene and Tropical Medicine	None-professional diplomas only available to physicians based in London and nurses/midwives (3–12 months) https://www.lshtm.ac.uk/study/courses/professional-development/professional-diplomas	None
	Pharmacists can have access to a short course (4 days) https://www.lshtm.ac.uk/study/courses/short-courses/travel-medicine	None
Liverpool School of Tropical Medicine	Travel Vaccination- Principles and Practice (5 weeks)	None
	Malaria prevention in Travel Health (3 weeks) http://www.lstmed.ac.uk/study/courses	None
Centre for Pharmacy Postgraduate Education	Travel health- understanding and supporting travellers' wellbeing https://www.cppe.ac.uk/programmes/1/travel-e-02/	Evidence for Royal Pharmaceutical Society Faculty framework https://www.rpharms.com/professional-development/faculty/about-the-faculty
National Pharmacy Association	Travel PGDs https://www.npa.co.uk/training/patient-group-directions/travel-pgd/	None
British Global Travel Health Association (BGTHA)	ABC of travel health https://www.abcoftravelhealth.com	None
National Travel Health Network and Centre (NaTHNaC)	Yellow training and clinic registration https://nathnacyfzone.org.uk	Accreditation to provide Yellow Fever vaccination and registration of clinic

Additionally an external representative body, the British Global Travel Health Association (BGTHA) has produced its own e-learning programme that is currently awaiting accreditation.

5. Future

The Association of British Travel Agents travel trends report [1] indicates that there is a growth in early bookings for 2018 holidays and people are travelling to destinations not visited before. In the summer of 2017 the UK government announced a review of cost controls throughout areas of the NHS. Amongst this was a proposal to remove all vaccines currently provided free of charge for travel (hepatitis A, typhoid, combined tetanus/diphtheria/polio, and cholera) from NHS supply. The NHS has since requested a feasibility study to be completed by Public Health England [7] on the complete removal of these vaccines and the subsequent impact on public health services. The findings are awaiting publication.

6. Discussion

Within the UK the changes in national legislation have provided wider and more extensive powers for pharmacists to supply POM medication. The term travel health is undefined and yet to be recognised by the General Medical Council as a medical speciality. The consequence is that a pharmacist can initiate a travel health service and the levels of service being offered can vary from the supply of antimalarial medication to specialists who have completed an extensive level of training. To become competent in travel health, pharmacist practitioners should consider the need to complete an independent prescribers course, a recognised formal qualification in travel health and membership to a medical Royal College. This has been accomplished by a small number of pharmacist practitioners,

Pharmacy **2018**, *6*, 64

however the practice of travel health without all of the additional skill sets, relies on the pharmacist to understand the limits of their competency when assessing and providing a clinical service.

As highlighted before, the supply function of POMs can be made using a PGD, however no mandatory training on the use is required to use these. The other supply function is using an independent prescriber that trains in a specific area of competency but are legally allowed to prescribe any POM. A consequence of this is that pharmacist independent prescribers can supply travel health medication without being specifically trained in the specialist clinical area.

The professional guidelines advise that independent prescribers should only practice within their competency and that PGDs are only used following specific training. Due to the complex nature of travel health a review is required of the supply provision and training and that should include arrangements for referral of complex patient cases to specialist pharmacists. The need of specialist, mandatory training is supported by the Faculty of Travel Medicine who have published a statement indicating that there is no licensing or checks on the level of care and that travellers are at risk [15].

By comparison in Alberta, Canada pharmacist provided travel health services are supplied by suitably trained pharmacists with basic life support skills and prescribing skills. The additional requirement is the completion of a formally recognised qualification in travel health, such as the Certificate of Knowledge of the International Society of Travel Medicine [16].

7. Conclusions

Travel health provision through UK community pharmacies is well advanced due to changes in national legislation. The supply of POM medications using PGD and independent prescriber services allows any pharmacist to privately supply travel health medication; however the minimum skill base to provide these services remains undefined and not legally required. To ensure the ongoing safety of travellers then the UK licensing authorities need to consider working with the specialist education providers to define minimum standards of competence for pharmacists. The formal training of advanced level services available to pharmacists is supplied through a single awarding institution, with other institutions selectively offering to medical practitioners and nurses only. To match the demand of pharmacist level travel health services more formally certified post-graduate courses in travel medicine would need to be made available. The future would indicate that with more people travelling there would be an increased demand on travel health services in the UK.

Conflicts of Interest: The author is an independent travel medicine specialist and has no conflicts of interest to disclose.

References

1. Association of British Travel Agents (ABTA). Travel Trends Report. 2018. Available online: https://abta. com/assets/uploads/general/ABTA_Travel_Trends_Report_2018.pdf (accessed on 12 March 2018).
2. Department of Health. *Health Service Circular 2000/026*; National Health Service Executive: London, UK, 2000.
3. Cook, R. A brief guide to the new supplementary prescribing. *Nurs. Times* **2002**, *98*, 26. [PubMed]
4. Department of Health. A Guide to Implementing Nurse and Pharmacist Independent Prescribing within the NHS in England. 2006. Available online: http://webarchive.nationalarchives.gov.uk/20130124072757/http: /www.dh.gov.uk/prod_consum_dh/groups/dh_digitalassets/@dh/@en/documents/digitalasset/dh_ 4133747.pdf (accessed on 12 March 2018).
5. NICE Pathways. Non-Medical Prescribing. 2018. Available online: https://bnf.nice.org.uk/guidance/non-medical-prescribing.html (accessed on 12 March 2018).
6. Statutory Instruments. *The Human Medicines Regulations*; No 1916; U.K. Government Statutory Instruments: London, UK, 2012.
7. Public Health England. Public Health England to consider removing travel vaccinations from NHS prescriptions. *Pharm. J.* **2017**, *299*, 7906. [CrossRef]
8. Valneva in Partnership (VIP). 2018. Available online: https://vip.valnevauk.com/home/?confirmedhcp=1 (accessed on 20 June 2018).

9.   Sukkar, E. Community Pharmacy in Great Britain 2016:   A Fragmented Market.   2016. Available online: https://www.pharmaceutical-journal.com/news-and-analysis/infographics/community-pharmacy-in-great-britain-2016-a-fragmented-market/20201210.article (accessed on 12 March 2018).

10.   Care Quality Commission. Healthcare Clinic. 2018. Available online: http://www.cqc.org.uk/what-we-do/services-we-regulate/find-healthcare-clinic (accessed on 19 March 2018).

11.   Care Quality Commission. Regulating Digital Healthcare Providers in Primary Care. 2017. Available online: http://www.cqc.org.uk/sites/default/files/20170303_pms-digital-healthcare_regulatory-uidance.pdf (accessed on 19 March 2018).

12.   Goodyer, L.; Devgi, V. A survey of Travel related medicines available through e-prescribing services in the UK. *J. BGTHA* **2014**, *24*, 53–55.

13.   Hind, C.; Bond, C.; Lee, A.; van Teijlingen, E. Travel medicine services from a community pharmacy: Evaluation of a pilot service. *Pharm. J.* **2008**, *281*, 625–632.

14.   Public Health England. National Minimum Standards and Core Curriculum for Immunisation Training for Registered Healthcare Practitioners. 2018. Available online: https://www.gov.uk/government/uploads/system/uploads/attachment_data/file/679824/Training_standards_and_core_curriculum_immunisation.pdf (accessed on 21 March 2018).

15.   Royal College of Physicians and Surgeons. Protecting the Health of Travellers from the UK and Ireland. 2015. Available online: https://rcpsg.ac.uk/documents/agm-and-elections/ftm/255-health-of-travellers/file (accessed on 26 June 2018).

16.   Houle, S.; Bascom, C.; Rosenthal, M. Clinical outcomes and satisfaction with a pharmacist—Managed travel clinic in Alberta, Canada. *Travel Med. Infect. Dis.* **2018**, *23*, 21–26. [CrossRef] [PubMed]

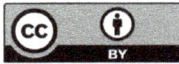

MDPI

St. Alban-Anlage 66

4052 Basel

Switzerland

Tel. +41 61 683 77 34

Fax +41 61 302 89 18

www.mdpi.com

Pharmacy Editorial Office

E-mail: pharmacy@mdpi.com

www.mdpi.com/journal/pharmacy

www.ingramcontent.com/pod-product-compliance
Lightning Source LLC
Chambersburg PA
CBHW051917210326
41597CB00033B/6175